FIND YOUR
INNER
SEX
GODDESS

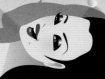

THIS IS A CARLTON BOOK

Text © 2004 Carlton Books Limited
Design and illustrations © 2006, 2013
Carlton Books Limited

This edition published in 2013 by
Carlton Books Limited
20 Mortimer Street
London W1T 3JW

10 9 8 7 6 5 4 3 2 1

This book was previously published
under the title *How to Be a Sex
Goddess* (2004).

A CIP catalogue record for this
book is available from the
British Library

ISBN 978-1-78097-445-3

Printed and bound in China

Illustrator: www.pinglet.com

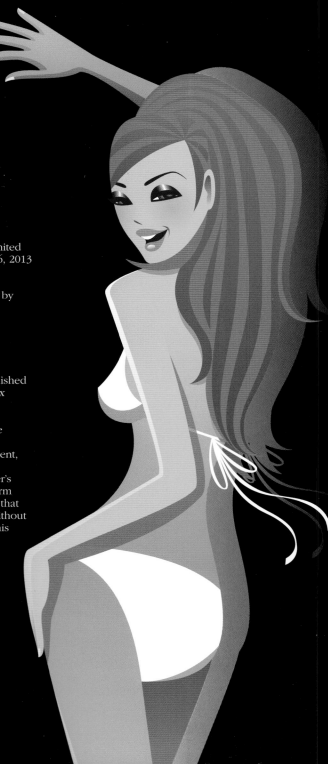

FIND YOUR INNER SEX GODDESS

LOUISE WESTON

CARLTON
BOOKS

CONTENTS

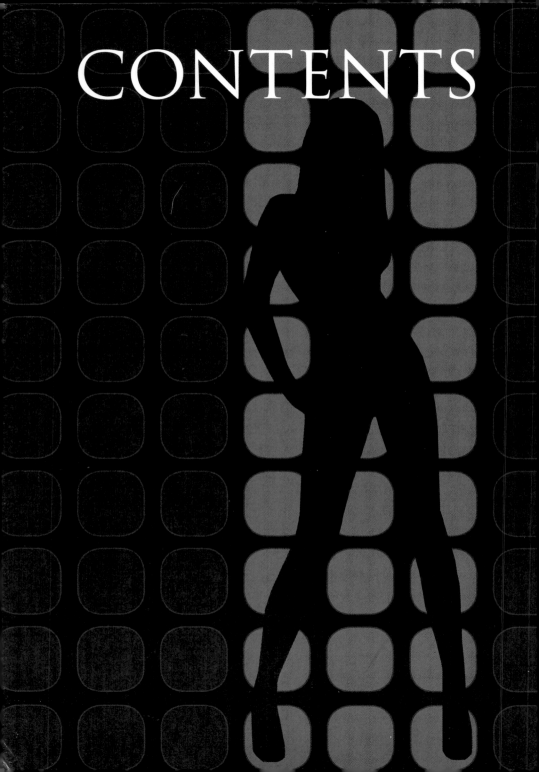

INTRODUCTION

It seems that modern life is full of instructions. Once it was considered enough simply to have your own teeth and get yourself out of bed in the morning without electric shock therapy. Nowadays, if you're not simultaneously whipping up the perfect sponge cake, negotiating a pay rise and dropping a dress size in a week, the self-help industry regards you as a dismal failure. So reading this book is not meant to be yet another stressful challenge. It is not a book that states that unless you take full account of the tips within you will fail the ensuing sex-goddess exam, or that if you don't immediately dump your existing wardrobe, develop a breathy purr and start sucking your finger whenever a man comes within a few metres of you, you'll never have satisfying sex. There's enough pressure on women already to be some kind of weird, inflatable fantasy figure – and the last thing I want to do is add to it.

So for our purposes, learning to be a sex goddess is simply learning to be a more confident, more self-loving version of who you already are. Most women, sadly, are riddled with doubts and insecurities, and we waste untold amounts of energy fretting about minuscule flaws and imagined defects, which no one else will ever notice or care about. The benefit of becoming a sex goddess is not that you will suddenly be able to perform a series of naked back flips into the bedroom before presenting your Kylie-sized butt for inspection. It's simply that you will feel sexier. Whether you're with the man you've been married to for twenty years, some bloke you met at the student disco last night or merely slumped on the sofa with your housemate, wondering whether fluoride in the water has killed all the eligible men in your town, it doesn't matter. Because if you feel sexy inside, you'll project sexy to the world, and the world will respond accordingly.

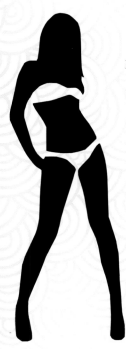

If you find some of the suggestions here embarrassing, or stupid, don't do them. If you feel like a prize prawn in stilettos, stick with flatties. If you look at the pictures and snort, 'Yeah, right! Like I'm really gonna do THAT after a hellish day at work', fair enough, pour yourself a nice glass of wine and watch TV instead. The kind of sex goddess you want to be is entirely up to you, not your man, your friends or even the authors of books.

'Ultimately, it all comes down to the old self-help classic: feeling good about yourself.'

And as far as I'm concerned, the one area of life where that matters most is sex. Who cares if you can't bake cakes? Who gives a stuff if you can't negotiate your way out of a paper bag or you don't know how to dress to minimize wide calves? Get a life. What matters is whether you can communicate with another person, whether you can show them what makes you feel great and make them feel great in return, and have the confidence in yourself that comes from believing you're truly desirable and loveable. That's what being a sex goddess is all about, everything else is just the icing on the shop-bought cake.

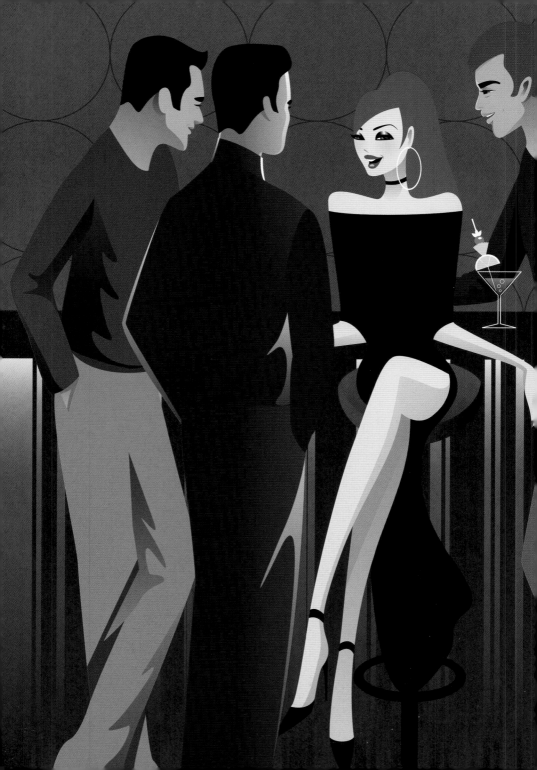

1 WHAT MAKES A SEX GODDESS?

'SEX APPEAL IS 50% WHAT YOU'VE GOT AND 50% WHAT PEOPLE THINK YOU'VE GOT.'

SOPHIA LOREN

HOW TO GET
SEX GODDESS ATTITUDE

I think you already know what I'm going to say first:
Anyone can be a sex goddess. You don't need butt-length blonde hair or hips that undulate like the Indian rope trick; you can be tiny or tall, fat or thin, beautiful or, well…, facially challenged. And you can still entrance men with your sexuality. For a truly sexy woman, men will move mountains, crawl over broken glass to the ends of the earth, rescue kittens stuck up redwood trees, hang themselves upside down across the Grand Canyon and generally make grade-A fools of themselves. All to be near you and, if they're lucky, to be in bed with you.

The most ordinary-looking women are capable of charming and disarming the most gorgeous men simply because they are sex goddesses in disguise. But their goddess-like status isn't conferred because of looks, or clothes or hairstyle, though all of these things can help.

The true difference between an attractive woman and a sex goddess is easy to define:

IT'S ATTITUDE.

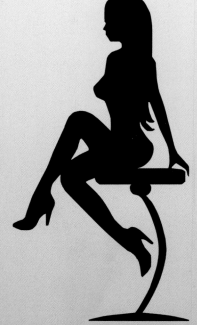

1 CONFIDENCE

A true sex goddess has confidence in herself. When a man compliments her on her body, she does not reply, 'Oh my God, no! You must be joking! I'm huge!'. She doesn't give men the chance to judge her and find her wanting by investing their opinions with too much power. If a man is rude or thoughtless, or insensitive, she walks away. She doesn't stick around hoping she'll be the one to change him. She knows exactly what she wants and, more importantly, she understands precisely what she needs from a sexual encounter or relationship. And if she's unlikely to be satisfied, she doesn't pursue it. In short, she knows she's gorgeous and that she deserves the best. This is not arrogance, it's pure self-belief. Basically, no one treats her badly – they wouldn't dare to.

2 GSOH

Sex goddesses have a sense of humour. Any number of women can be beautiful: they can put on a bedroom performance like Ginger Rogers on speed and they can gaze adoringly into his eyes. But without the vital spark that comes from experience, native wit and the innate understanding of other people, which makes up a sense of humour, the whole encounter can be as dead as a night with an inflatable doll. Sex goddesses avoid constantly cracking jokes – a barrage of gags can kill any sex session in seconds. However, they know exactly when to break any tension in the atmosphere with a quip – like when the condom's just pinged off for the third time.

3 RELAXATION

So what's the final key to identifying a sex goddess? She's relaxed, so comfortable with herself that she listens properly to others and talks easily. A neurotic, flapping woman will never be a goddess – she's far too concerned with what other people think of her, forever panicking about the impression she's making and the clothes she's wearing. She displays all the nervy body language of a pure-bred whippet, fiddling with her hair and picking at her nails. An unrelaxed person makes everyone else tense. In any social – or sexual – situation, a real sex goddess is completely chilled out, sensual in her touches, calm in her own skin and as relaxed as a cat lounging by the fireside.

INNER AND OUTER BEAUTY

The bad news is that about 0.1 per cent of us are natural sex goddesses. However, the up side of this is that the other 99.9 per cent can learn those skills and reach sex-goddess level without the help of plastic surgery, hair dye, liposuction or ten hours a day at the gym. Of course you can do all that if you really want to, but at the end of the day you may run the risk of being a very fit, very slim neurotic. No man will want to go to bed with you just in case you turn into a mental Bunny Boiler the morning after.

Sex goddesses don't seem as though they're trying too hard. If you turn up at a party with a mahogany tan, surgically honed limbs, a cloud of peroxide hair and a dress the size of Barbie's hanky, for sure, some men will want to sleep with you. But they'll also assume you're desperate for attention and very insecure – and they'll be keen to call you a cab straight after sex to whisk you out of their lives before you get too troublesome. This is not the effect you desire, trust me.

That's not to say that physical appearance counts for nothing: it does. But without wishing to sound like your mother (while being fully aware that I probably do), you need to realize that almost always sex-goddess beauty comes from 'Making the Most of What You've Got'. Not from copying Cheryl Cole's hair, going on the same diet as Jennifer Aniston, doing your eyeliner like your best mate or buying insane, hillbilly clothes because a magazine said they were in vogue. Fashion is not the same thing as style, and every aspiring sex goddess should have that simple fact tattooed over her heart.

> ## *'It's all about dressing appropriately, highlighting the good bits and minimizing the bad.'*

Sex goddess beauty also relies on you accepting your age. While you can certainly enhance your looks – I'm all for wrinkle-defying creams, root touch-ups, eyebrow-plucking and the like – actively refuting the calendar is a dangerous game to play. Dressing too young for your age – 'mutton dressed as lamb' – is a terrible style to favour. All it does is highlight the vast discrepancy between teeny-weeny teenage garments and your somewhat larger limbs and boobs. When choosing clothes, any woman over 25 should ask herself, 'Would the average 15-year-old wear this?' If the answer is 'yes', then think very carefully indeed before buying.

Of course, it cuts both ways, and the under-45s should not be caught out stomping around in 1980s-style piecrust collars and badly cut sensible skirts – nor should the over-45s if they want to continue to be goddesses. Be wary of fashion trends that never really worked the first time around. I'm thinking sickly yellow, dungarees (overalls) and pinafore dresses. By all means, keep current and move with the times, but know yourself enough to let your unique personality shine through and select according to what works well for you.

DRESS TO IMPRESS

Get help if you have the colour sense of a drunken bat and the innate style of Marilyn Manson. Like Bridget Jones's mother, get your 'colours done' to find out whether you're suited to brights or neutrals and edit your wardrobe accordingly. Alternatively, consider a capsule wardrobe of separates that you know work for you. Ask a friend to go shopping and beg her (or him – gay men are honest shopping companions) to be brutally frank. It's simple really. If you have good legs, buy a well-tailored short skirt. Lumpy knees but a great bust? Wear trousers with low-necked tops. Spend as much as you can afford on well-cut clothes in natural, sensual fabrics. They hang better, feel nicer and they make you want to swish around, murmuring, 'Because I'm worth it'.

A sex goddess knows it's better to have three stunning outfits rather than sixty different tops and skirts that are inexpensive but fall apart at the first wash. You wouldn't shampoo your hair with dishwashing liquid and still expect to look good, so why wear badly made clothes and expect to feel sexy? Being poor, by the way, is no excuse. You can buy second-hand designer clothes from charity shops, or go to 75-per-cent-off or sample sales. There are many women who have nurtured the talent of never buying 'retail'. I, however, do spend a lot on shoes. Every aspiring sex goddess needs at least one indulgence, and Marc Jacobs footwear is mine.

YOUR CROWNING GLORY

The next thing you need is a decent haircut (and/or colour). Not because it will attract men (most straight men wouldn't know John Frieda from John Cleese), but simply because a great cut makes you feel fantastic, so you project confidence, sex appeal and self-belief wherever you go.

Again, go to the best salon you can afford and don't be bullied into trying something 'directional'. Women who mumble, 'Well, I don't know really, what do you think?' to some scissors-wielding megalomaniac are just asking for trouble. Take charge and show the hairstylists pictures of styles you admire. Be persistent and demand the kind of cut that shapes your face, falls easily into place without an hour of straightening irons and styling products every morning, and looks as though a man could run his fingers through it without getting them tangled up in style complexities.

The best hair colour for you entirely depends on the rest of your colouring. You can dye it any shade you want, but if your skin tone doesn't match your hair, you'll look more Edward Scissorhands than a glossy-tressed beauty. Only go blonde if you're not deathly pale and your natural hair colour isn't so dark your root regrowth becomes an issue every three days. Red hair doesn't suit girls with pink complexions, but brown does. Black hair is not a good look for most women; it's deeply draining, so only do it if you've got olive skin. And 'fun' colours like blue and pink only work if you've got the fun dress sense to match – bright green hair and a Donna Karan suit looks more like a practical joke than a style.

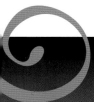

MAKING UP ISN'T SO HARD TO DO

Then there's make-up. It goes without saying that a face resembling Cleopatra's death mask is not terribly attractive. Like men with heavy beards, women with strong make-up always look as if they've got something to hide. Acne, hideous scars, teeny piggy little eyes… while none of this may be true, passers-by will be suspicious because you've done such a number on yourself. Again, when it comes to make-up, the key words are 'relaxation' and 'confidence'.

A good moisturizer is vital. Buy the best you can, otherwise your foundation will soon become patchy and you'll look like a dog that's rolled in mud. Foundation should be as pale and as close to your skin tone as possible – never try to give yourself a tan with it, you'll just look freakish. Your desert-island essentials are: blusher (use a tiny amount to avoid enormous 1980s stripes down your face); eyebrow pencil (well-shaped brows make the face – if you need proof, look at before and after photos of Elizabeth Hurley); brown or black mascara to open up your eyes and make you look interested even when you're not; and the most essential product of all, a lipstick or tinted gloss to keep the focus on your pouty, kiss-worthy lips. You might also want to apply powder to prevent your skin shining too much. Other than that, forget it. Cosmetic fads are so-called for a reason: they don't suit anyone. Just because some stunning 16-year-old occasionally gets away with it on a catwalk, it doesn't mean you can too (which is why green mascara is always in the half-price basket at the pharmacy).

THE BODY BEAUTIFUL

Often it's body image that stops many a wannabe sex goddess in her tracks. Convinced that unless she is the size of a Chihuahua she'll never be sexy, she hides herself in huge sweaters, hunches over to conceal her stomach and generally creeps about. So of course she's not alluring. I know no one will believe me (and sometimes I have a hard time convincing myself, particularly after the second crème brûlée), but here's the truth: Men Fancy All Shapes and Sizes of Women. Some even think sex with a skinny girl is like riding a bicycle. Others find flab frightening. Some like their women medium sized, others prefer petite, while still more love tall girls. Basically, as Osgood says at the end of the movie, *Some Like It Hot*, 'Well, nobody's perfect.' And if they are, they're probably fantastically dull people who would rather spend a spare hour pounding away on a treadmill than drinking fine wine with friends, losing themselves in a great book or having fabulous sex for hours on end.

'Well, nobody's perfect.'

What it comes down to is not, 'Am I thin/toned/shapely enough?', but 'Do I accept and like what I am enough?' If the answer is 'no', then ask yourself why. Those who reply, 'Because I'm a disgusting person who's weak and a failure' should forget the gym for now and head straight for therapy without passing go. Others who say, 'Because I've put on weight and I feel a bit less energetic and attractive' can soon sort themselves out with a bit of willpower by eating less and exerting themselves more. But a word of warning: there's nothing goddess-like about banging on endlessly about your diet. Your friends, your colleagues and your men won't care what you think about Dr Atkins or South Beach. All that matters to them is that you like and accept yourself as you are. Telling your date you've lost 2.2 kg (5 lb) in a week by only eating cabbage soup will not entice him. He'll simply gain a hideous image of you crouched like some madwoman over a pot of bubbling green scum, and he'll wonder why it's so important to you that you deprive yourself of all pleasure – not to mention risk the nasty side effects.

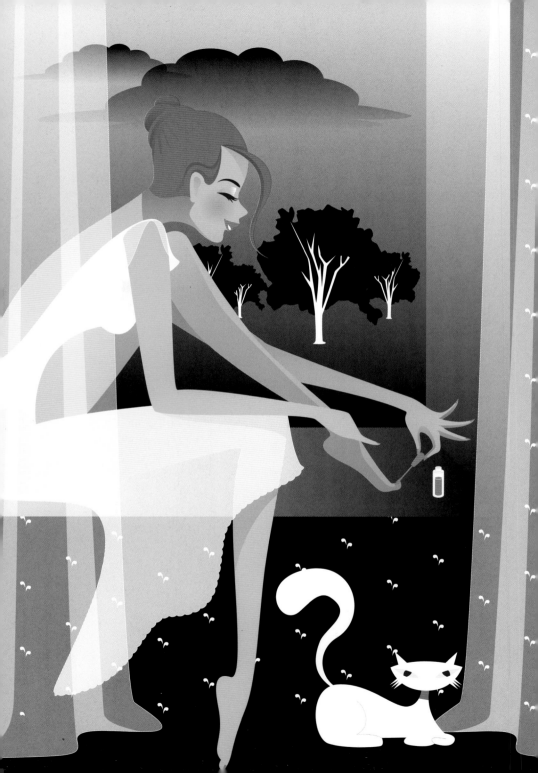

If you are trying to lose weight, keep quiet and get on with it. The no-carbs-in-the-evening system works for me and avoids the pangs of complete carbohydrate withdrawal: you don't get hungry, you lose weight and you can still drink alcohol. And if, like me, you find the gym a torture chamber of mindless pain, seek out something that's more enjoyable for you that burns calories, whether it's dancing, gardening, swimming, sex or skating, and do it three times a week. Before starting any exercise routine seek medical advice, especially if you are overweight, take medication or suffer from any health problems.

If you decide life's too short for all this deprivation and exhaustion, fine. You just have to make the decision to like yourself the way you are and take a solemn vow never to ask a sexual partner if he thinks you're too fat. If he answers 'yes', you'll be devastated, and should he say 'no', you'll decide he's just being nice. So deal with it yourself.

GROOMED FOR SUCCESS

As far as appearance goes, the true sex goddess wears whatever she wants and looks how she desires – but she is always groomed. By 'groomed' I don't mean prissy pearl necklaces and velvet headbands like some society gal; I mean clean and fresh – everywhere from her hair to her teeth, her hands to her toes – and looking as though she'd be nice to touch. She's clean, sexy and smells nice. Body lotion that gives skin a sheen is more goddess-like than dry, scaly patches, and buffed or varnished toenails are more appealing than yellowing claws, while shaved legs and a trimmed bikini line will give you more confidence than a sprawling Teutonic bush that escapes from your Lycra. You know you could strip off at a moment's notice and all would be in order. A real sex goddess looks as though she cares about herself, and you should, too.

If you don't love and respect yourself, why should anyone else? Present an image that's like a sack of washing and, honey, you'll get treated like one. It's sad but true: first impressions count.

SEX GODDESS LINE-UP

OK, so you've got all the basics. You're thinking more about attitude, you might buy a nice pair of trousers that flatter your butt. Hell, you always clean your teeth. Now it's time for a little inspiration – a quick glance at the women who've really got the whole sex-goddess thing going. Of course, all these goddesses have had bad days and suffered PMT (PMS) or stomach bugs; all occasionally looked a mess. But they had, or have, attitude and they knew how to work what they had. So pick out your favourite sex goddess and be inspired.

JOSEPHINE BAKER

In the 1920s, Josephine Baker was the first black dancer to star in the Folies Bergère and danced the charleston sporting only coloured feathers round her hips. The 'Black Venus' reportedly received 1,500 marriage proposals in her lifetime. A World War II resistance fighter, she once escaped down Goering's laundry chute, and was decorated for her bravery. After the war she adopted eleven children of different races and religions, and devoted her life to fighting racism.

LAUREN BACALL

Bacall made a virtue of her man-deep voice, knew exactly
how to whistle and when she was 73 she was selected as
one of the fifty most beautiful people in the world by *People*
magazine. She married Humphrey Bogart, her co-star in *To
Have and Have Not*, though commented, 'I never believed
marriage was a lasting institution… I thought that to be
married for five years was to be married forever.' Cool as.

MAE WEST

From the age of five Mae West starred in vaudeville. By 14,
she was known as the 'Baby Vamp' – and a little later she
wrote her own play, *Sex*, which landed her in jail for ten days
on obscenity charges. Famous as much for her wit as her
looks – 'I used to be Snow White, but I drifted' – she enjoyed
writing innuendo-packed scripts to slip past the moral codes
of the time. West mocked repressive society, and did much to
open up communication about female sexuality. As she once
said, 'Goodness had nothing to do with it.'

RAQUEL WELCH

Raquel still possesses the face and the figure to stop a six-lane
highway – seen to best effect in the fur bikini of *One Million
Years B.C.* Four husbands, backstage feuds and court cases
have made her the ultimate diva – and she still doesn't suffer
fools. 'Please yourself and follow your own instincts – only
then can you be successful. You become more satisfied, and
when you are, other people will tend to be satisfied by what
you do.'

MARLENE DIETRICH

Legs to die for and a heartbreaking voice were Marlene's trademarks as the 'Blue Angel'. But in 1935, Adolf Hitler demanded that the famous German actress return to the Fatherland. Dietrich, an anti-Nazi, refused, and all her films were banned from Germany. She became a US citizen and during World War II she devoted most of her energy to entertaining allied troops with the sentimental ballad 'Lili Marlene'. Brave and beautiful, she was the epitome of the glamorous nightclub singer.

LILLIE LANGTRY

The twentieth century's first celebrity sex goddess, the stunning Langtry took many lovers, including Prince Albert. Her beauty inspired both writers and artists, she advertised Pears soap and her portrait became an early pin-up postcard. Her view was that 'men are born to be slaves'. When Albert complained, 'I've spent enough on you to buy a battleship,' she replied, 'You've spent enough in me to float one.' Not just a pretty face…

CATHERINE DENEUVE

France's best export, Deneuve combines elegance, beauty and intelligence. Her roles as a prostitute in Luis Buñuel's *Belle de Jour* and a killer in Roman Polanski's *Repulsion* propelled her to global fame, though she waited until 1992 for an Oscar nomination (for *Indochine*). Married to goddess-collectors Roger Vadim and David Bailey, Deneuve is also the mother of Marcello Mastroianni's child and the muse of Yves Saint Laurent. Today, Deneuve still drives men wild.

ELIZABETH TAYLOR

Famed for her violet eyes, Elizabeth Taylor was one of the most beautiful actresses in the movies, and her charity work for AIDS keeps her twinkling at goddess level. From the child star in *National Velvet* to alcoholic Martha in *Who's Afraid of Virginia Woolf?* she has mesmerized generations of viewers with her seductive screen presence and awe-inspiring talent. Her personal life alone is worth many biographies, while her tempestuous love affair and marriages with Richard Burton are positively legendary. Then there's the diamonds, the millions, oh, and the seven husbands…. 'My mother says I didn't open my eyes for eight days after I was born – but when I did, the first thing I saw was an engagement ring. I was hooked.'

BRIGITTE BARDOT

A model by 15, the beautiful BB became a 1960s icon when she moved into French films, starring in such sex-kitten roles as Juliet in Roger Vadim's *And God Created Woman*. At 18 she married Vadim (who seems to have had some magic goddess-magnet) and five years later she divorced him. She recorded a number of songs in the 1960s and 1970s, but fame never suited her, despite the adulation for her French chic, her cool and her beauty. She retired from the silver screen in 1975, but that didn't stop the paparazzi and legions of fans from pursuing this living legend. She did her own thing in the end, becoming a vocal spokesperson for animal rights and starting up her successful Brigitte Bardot Foundation for the cause. She remains a goddess because she doesn't care now, and she never did.

SOPHIA LOREN

Sophia grew up in the slums of Naples, but her jaw-dropping
looks and curvy body were a swift passport to movie success.
She won an Oscar in 1961 for *La Ciociara* (*Two Women*), married
director Carlo Ponti, twenty-two years her senior, (a marriage
she annulled to save him from bigamy charges) and became
close friends with Cary Grant. She also served eighteen days in
an Italian prison for tax evasion – hey, even goddesses get their
maths wrong. Loren is crowned a goddess for her style, her looks
and most of all, her famous quote, which every aspiring goddess
should remember: 'Sex appeal is 50 per cent what you've got and
50 per cent what people think you've got.'

HALLE BERRY

Striking a serious plaudit for black sex goddesses everywhere,
Halle won her Oscar for *Monster's Ball* in 2002 – the first-ever
won by an African American – and the world wept right along
with her. She's gorgeous, feisty and so dedicated to her career
that she refused to bathe prior to her role as a crack addict in
Spike Lee's *Jungle Fever*. She's also a Bond girl and ex-beauty
pageant winner. But mostly, Halle's a goddess because, as
she put it herself, clutching her Oscar, 'It's for every nameless,
faceless woman of colour that now has a chance – because the
door tonight has been opened.'

MARILYN MONROE

Not just a sex goddess, but *the* sex goddess. A combination of sexual allure, wit, charm and vulnerability made Marilyn the ultimate pin-up. Men wanted her; women wanted to look like her. She experienced it all – the orphanage upbringing, the untimely death, the marriages and affairs with all the gods of the time, including Joe DiMaggio, Arthur Miller, JFK and Frank Sinatra. As well as her staggering prettiness and hourglass figure, she was entirely at ease with her sexuality. 'Sex is a part of nature. I go along with nature,' she once said. And the entire nation knew what she wore in bed – Chanel No. 5. From her platinum-blonde hair to the tips of her toes, the woman was a true goddess.

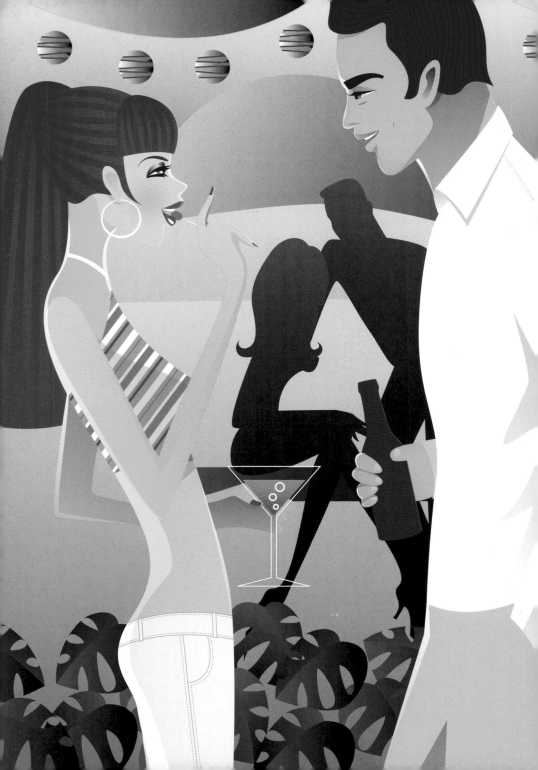

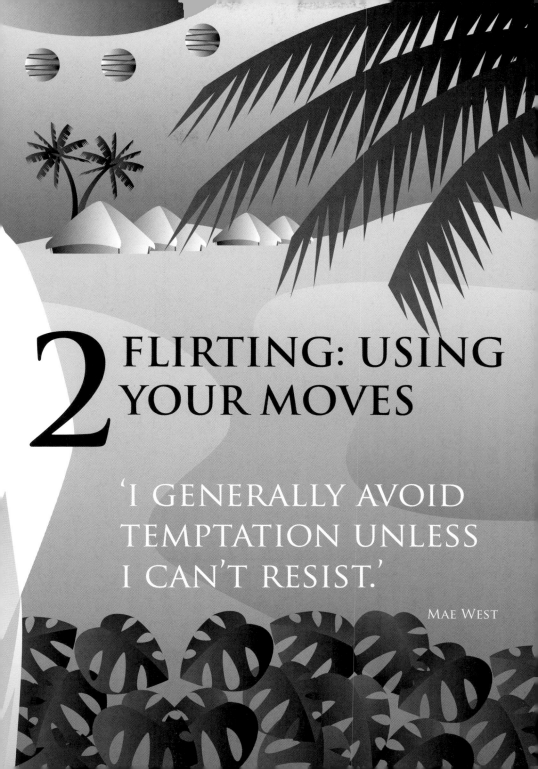

2 FLIRTING: USING YOUR MOVES

'I GENERALLY AVOID TEMPTATION UNLESS I CAN'T RESIST.'

MAE WEST

STAGE ONE: MEETING

So you're in a bar, a gym, an art gallery or any other normal venue where male and female strangers congregate. You could even be in court, but if you're the defendant, try to save your hot moves for later. You spot a male god, whom you think would go nicely with you, a goddess. But he's not looking at you, so what do you do? Avoid anything cheesy such as sending over a drink – he'll assume you're crazy about him, and whatever relationship transpires from this, you'll always be on the back foot, having initiated the chase. Ideally, you want him to think that he spotted you first. Okay, it goes against all feminist principles and it's a dismal throwback, but the truth is that most men like to do the chasing, at least initially. So fixate your eyes on him. It's weird but true that everyone knows when they're being stared at, and it's probably something to do with our Stone-Age defence system, when the forests were full of people trying to kill the juicy mammoth first. As he turns to locate the source of the staring, flick your eyes away quickly.

Anyone can flirt but the truth is, not everyone can do it effectively. We all know how to toss our hair and how to run our tongues over our lips suggestively, but unless it's carefully done there's a very real risk of looking like a drag queen rather than the subtle creature of mystery you were intending. Good flirting is subtle. A true sex goddess is an excellent flirt, but she never appears desperate. There's a world of difference between body language that eases communication and opens up interesting sensual possibilities, and the kind that shrieks, 'I haven't been laid for six months, what are you going to do about it?' As a sex goddess wannabe, obviously, you'll be aiming for the former.

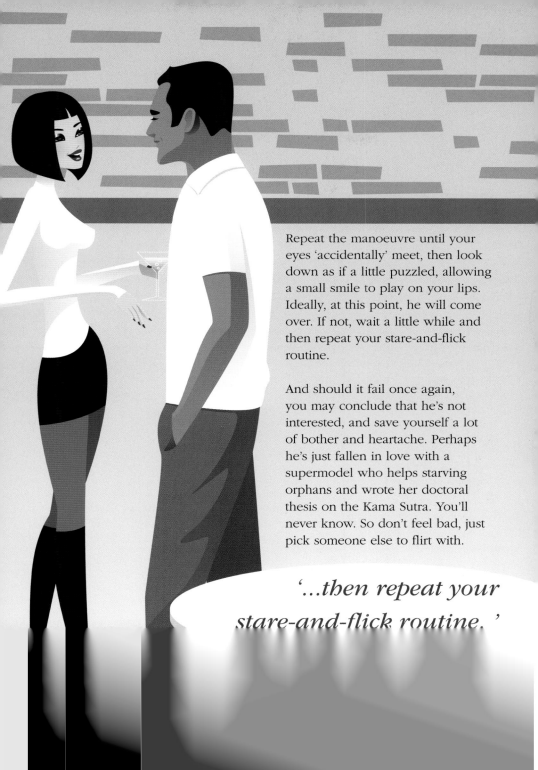

Repeat the manoeuvre until your eyes 'accidentally' meet, then look down as if a little puzzled, allowing a small smile to play on your lips. Ideally, at this point, he will come over. If not, wait a little while and then repeat your stare-and-flick routine.

And should it fail once again, you may conclude that he's not interested, and save yourself a lot of bother and heartache. Perhaps he's just fallen in love with a supermodel who helps starving orphans and wrote her doctoral thesis on the Kama Sutra. You'll never know. So don't feel bad, just pick someone else to flirt with.

'...then repeat your stare-and-flick routine. '

STAGE TWO: TALKING

Let's assume you've found your fellow flirtee and he's now standing in front of you. A true sex goddess won't get all touchy-feely right away – that's so obvious you may as well lift up your top and ask him to sign your breasts. You want to create the impression that you're quite interested in what he has to say and you certainly don't find him unattractive, without actually making it clear that given half a chance, you'd lock him away in your bedroom and never let him go.

One cunning way of doing this is to create a shared world for the two of you. A line such as 'Is it just me or does everyone else in here look like the cast of *The O.C.*?' (or *The Walking Dead*, or *The Sopranos*, depending on where you are) will suggest that he is the only person like you in the whole place, which is a very intimate suggestion without actually being a statement of intent. You are also creating a feeling that the rest of the world is dropping away and there's only the two of you left.

Smile more than you normally would – not goofy, tail-wagging grins, just slow, almost-reluctant smiles that imply you didn't really intend to smile but you're having such a good time you just can't help it. You can also afford to laugh once or twice at his jokes, but make sure you have an appealing laugh. Many a man has been terrified off by a woman's donkey-like hee-hawing or her nerve-jangling shriek. A warm, low murmur of amusement is a lot better than a snorting cackle. Pretend you're on the radio, and ask yourself whether listeners would leap up to retune the dial in horror or laugh along with you.

A good flirt is never nervous; confidence is the key to successful flirting. So when he compliments you on your appearance, don't reply, 'No, I don't – I look a mess, actually. I'm only wearing it because my girlfriend borrowed the top I really wanted to wear.' Instead, say, 'Thanks, you don't look so bad yourself.' Gabbling inanely and offering way too much information are also the enemies of the successful flirt. Hold back and offer your thoughts on a strictly need-to-know basis. Topics to avoid talking about as you flirt include: politics, illness, depression, your ex, his ex, money, how long you've been single and why you're a disaster with men. Don't bombard him with probing questions about his life and work – he'll feel as if he's being interviewed. A simple exchange of witty banter is all that's required at this stage.

'A good flirt is never nervous; confidence is the key to successful flirting.'

BODY LANGUAGE

If talking is the bread, body language is the meaty filling in your flirtation sandwich. Actions speak louder than words, and while what you're saying can be perfectly innocuous, what you're doing as you say it makes all the difference. The main thing, of course, is lots and lots of eye contact. Hold his gaze, look down and glance up occasionally from under your lashes – but don't do it too often and make sure you never look over his shoulder as if scanning for something (or someone) more interesting in the distance. If you really are attracted to him, your pupils will dilate. This has a stunning effect on men. In experiments, men consistently picked out women with larger pupils as being more attractive because it's a sign of sexual excitement and therefore, willingness. If you'd like your pupils to dilate and you're not sure his looks are enough on their own, just think about the last really good sex you had – even if it was by yourself. And don't look at bright lights, or your pupils will shrivel so fast you'll look like a heroin addict.

While overt touching can be too much straight away, there's plenty of moves you can make that will draw his attention to all the right areas. Most important is the angle of your body. Stand or sit facing him directly, so your attention can be focused entirely on each other. If you cross your legs, point your upper foot towards him – pointing away suggests a desire to turn your entire body away from the conversation. If they're not crossed, point your knees towards him and if you're standing, lean in slightly. When you speak, even if the place isn't that loud, position yourself close to his ear. Shouting is not intimate, but a close, low-voiced comment is. By talking more quietly, as well, you'll encourage him to lean further towards you so he doesn't miss a moment of your sparkling conversation.

To draw his attention to your best features, idly trail your fingers along your necklace if you have a fine bust, or rest your hand on your knee if your legs are great. If you've got a lovely J.Lo or Beyoncé butt, remember you're not a baboon – you'll just have to wait for him to notice it.

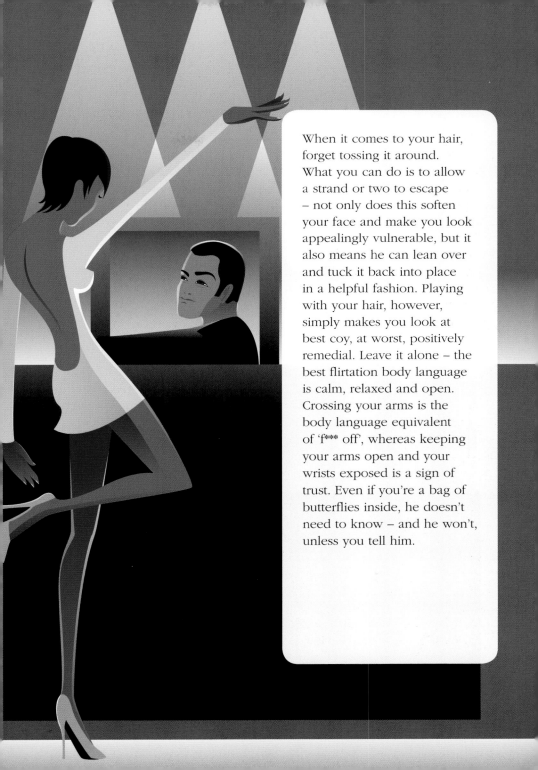

When it comes to your hair, forget tossing it around. What you can do is to allow a strand or two to escape – not only does this soften your face and make you look appealingly vulnerable, but it also means he can lean over and tuck it back into place in a helpful fashion. Playing with your hair, however, simply makes you look at best coy, at worst, positively remedial. Leave it alone – the best flirtation body language is calm, relaxed and open. Crossing your arms is the body language equivalent of 'f*** off', whereas keeping your arms open and your wrists exposed is a sign of trust. Even if you're a bag of butterflies inside, he doesn't need to know – and he won't, unless you tell him.

TOUCHING HIM

Once you're at ease with each other, and flirting has progressed from hair-smoothing and knee-pointing to the point where you're both aware that you like each other, you can start to touch him, lightly and sensually, to make your intentions perfectly clear. Not all over – you're a goddess, not a Cuban hooker – just light brushes with your fingertips to indicate that you really quite like him.

A quick touch of the knee to emphasize what you're saying is a good starting point. You can also use the old brushing-invisible-fluff-off-the-shirt trick, but go carefully with this one or there's a significant danger you'll remind him of his mother and he'll fear you're about to spit on a hanky and wipe his face clean. A simple lean-forward-and-flick motion is fine. But don't start grooming him like a female gibbon picking fleas off her mate.

Another intimate little move is to pick up his wrist and turn it so you can see the time on his watch – although avoid doing this while he's holding a drink. If you smoke, you can make use of the old film noir technique where you hold his hand to steady the flame, while looking upwards into his eyes; this is pretty full-on, so should only be used when definite attraction has already been stated. Don't try the old trick of blowing a stream of smoke in his face, though – it's really not pleasant.

Forget too corny and creaky manoeuvres such as
'palm reading' – it's as transparent as a polished
aquarium. Also avoid the weary, 'I seem to have
something in my eye', *Brief Encounter* plan,
although, admittedly, it worked a little too well
for Celia Johnson. You can make your intentions
perfectly clear by touching his forearm or the soft
skin above his elbow as you talk (ideally performed
as if you're barely aware of what you're doing,
simply implying that you're physically drawn to him
on some subconscious level). Or lightly squeeze his
hand during a moment of particular emphasis in the
conversation. Of course, as all these small touches
and subtle manoeuvres go on, he will almost
certainly be touching and flirting back with you –
the only difference being that, as a sex goddess,
you'll be doing it better.

*'…just light brushes
with your fingertips
indicate that you like him.'*

ANTI-FLIRTING

A sex goddess seldom finds herself in a situation she'd rather avoid because she has the tactics to extricate herself before it all goes wrong. Many untrained sex goddesses, however, make the mistake of being too encouraging to men who should by rights be squatting on lily pads, secreting poison. Not because they want to lure these creepy individuals, but simply because they don't know how to get rid of them. Luckily there are ways of repelling men without causing them to become offensive. It's just a matter of creating a shield around yourself, which they cannot pass, try as they might.

'It's just a matter of creating a shield around yourself, which they cannot pass.'

Anti-flirting begins with no eye contact. As you refuse that drink, avoid looking into his eyes. Everyone knows the eyes are the pathway to your soul and offer instant access to all your feelings of guilt, embarrassment and desire to make everyone like you. Truth is, you have no need to feel guilty – you didn't ask him to approach you, and you owe him nothing. The whole encounter is his responsibility; all you need to do is get rid of him. A goddess knows that not everyone has to like her – the only people whose opinion matters are the ones she likes.

If you are positioned near him, angle your body away from him. If you feel you must talk to him, make your answers brief. And if he has the nerve to make physical contact with you, slide out immediately from his touch – never give him the impression that he is permitted access to your body. Forget the classic victim's excuse of 'I didn't want to offend him'. Ask a nearby member of staff to remove him, or a sympathetic male to help out – and if there really is no one suitable around, invent a jealous boyfriend and predict his imminent return. You know all about not accepting drinks you haven't seen poured, not leaving a stranger in charge of your wine while you go to the bathroom and all that, don't you?

Of course you may know the creepy guy. Maybe he works in your office, he's working on your house or he lives next door… in which case you need to spell it out. You could also ask a male relative or friend to tell him to leave you alone.

Be careful not to send mixed messages. You may be agreeing to a drink because he seems lonely, but he may read your gesture as 'I want you, Tiger'. So watch it. Goddess or not, any sensible woman will never put herself in the path of danger that she can reasonably avoid.

LONG-TERM FLIRTING

Of course, in any serious relationship, you're not always going to be flirting like Bogie and Bacall over breakfast:

'You know how to whistle, don't you?'
'What? Why are you always asking me stupid
questions when I'm trying to read the paper?'

Naturally there are obstacles to the sort of flirtatious exchange you enjoyed when you first met, and that is an entirely normal part of the evolution of a relationship. You can, however, discover ways to 'sex it up' between you with a subtlety and humour you both will enjoy. To re-inject flirting with your long-time love, though, you're going to have to make a bit of an effort. However sex goddess-like you are, it's probably not going to happen in your home, surrounded by kids, bills, or with the TV blaring and the washing machine clunking. You need to go out on a date again to remind yourselves that you are, actually, a god and goddess – you simply got sidetracked from your true purpose by domesticity for a while. Here's your chance to rekindle those lovely moments of your early flirtation.

Choose a nicely lit hotel bar or restaurant and do not, under any circumstances, be tempted to meet up with friends at any stage of the evening. That's really not the point. Dress up, arrive separately and make a pact beforehand that you will not talk about the kids or work worries, or how much the loft conversion is going to cost. You have to make time to be romantic.

It's not going to happen by accident. And you don't need a fancy restaurant. You can have just as great an experience shopping for a luxurious dinner for two and cooking it together, or pack a picnic and whisk yourselves off to a lovely park or riverbank. It's also nice to share the stuff that interests you. The aim is to remind yourselves of what attracted you to each other at first before real life crept in, so keep the conversation light, sprinkled with wit and charm, and intersperse your nuggets of banter with plenty of hand-stroking and gazing into each other's eyes. If you feel this is all a bit contrived, take the pressure off by just going to the movies. But while you're there, if you don't want to snuggle up together in public, at least hold hands. You know how to hold hands, don't you? You just put your palms together and squeeze.

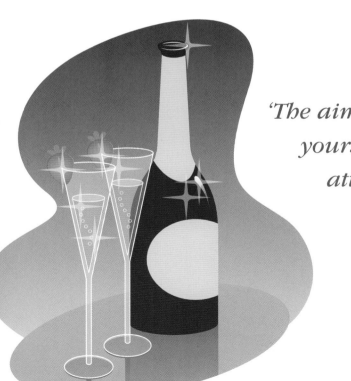

'The aim is to remind yourselves of what attracted you to each other.'

TOP TEN FLIRT TRICKS TO REMEMBER

1. Maintain eye contact but make sure you smile at the same time, or else you'll look like a crazy stalker.

2. Look down then up at him as if sneaking a quick glance – very sexy.

3. Raise your eyebrows and smile when you're impressed with what he's telling you.

4. Don't reveal too much about yourself – let him ask first.

5. Lean in to speak directly into his ear.

6. Sway to the music – most people suspect that sensual dancers are great in bed.

7. Don't bitch about other women or you'll look petty and insecure.

8. Accept compliments easily – never argue that he's wrong about what he thinks of you.

9. Brush your fingertips lightly across his arm or knee during conversation.

10. Keep it light – make jokes, not serious points about the world.

GOOD REASONS FOR FLIRTING

BAD REASONS FOR FLIRTING

There are good and bad reasons for flirting. Sex goddesses only flirt for the right ones. These include:

1. Because you fancy him.

2. Because you're making yourself feel good, but only when he's doing the same thing and there's no intent on either side.

3. Because you've been together for ages and flirting cheers things up no end.

4. You're also allowed to flirt with close male friends, so long as they don't have overly jealous girlfriends, just to get in a bit of practice.

1. To make your boyfriend jealous.

2. To try to recapture an ex who dumped you because you hope it might lead to sex that will make you feel loved, albeit briefly.

3. To annoy girls you don't like by flirting with their boyfriends or husbands, right in front of them.

Beware: nine times out of ten, bad-reason flirting will backfire on you. The ex will sleep with you and you'll wake up re-dumped and humiliated, or you'll gain a nasty reputation among the girls for being a cocktease and a woman who can't be trusted. Your boyfriend will go and snog someone else in retaliation, or you'll have a massive row. So when you are about to start flirting, stop and ask yourself what your intentions are first. If in doubt, stop batting those eyelashes at once.

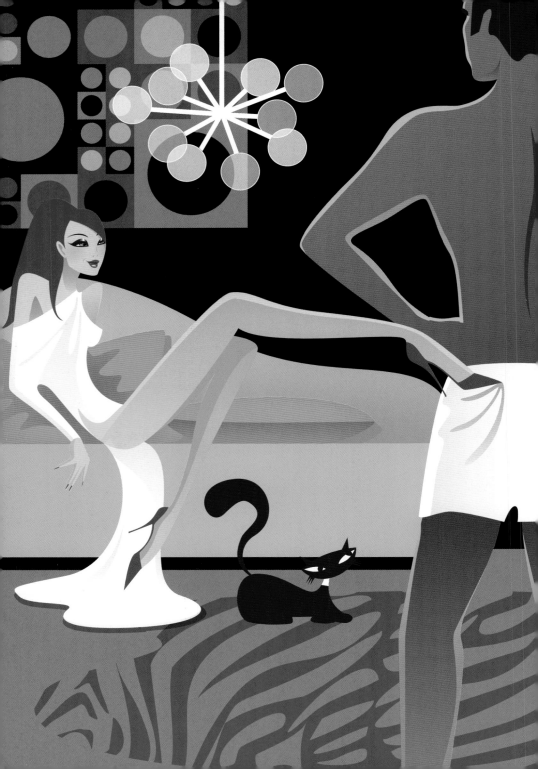

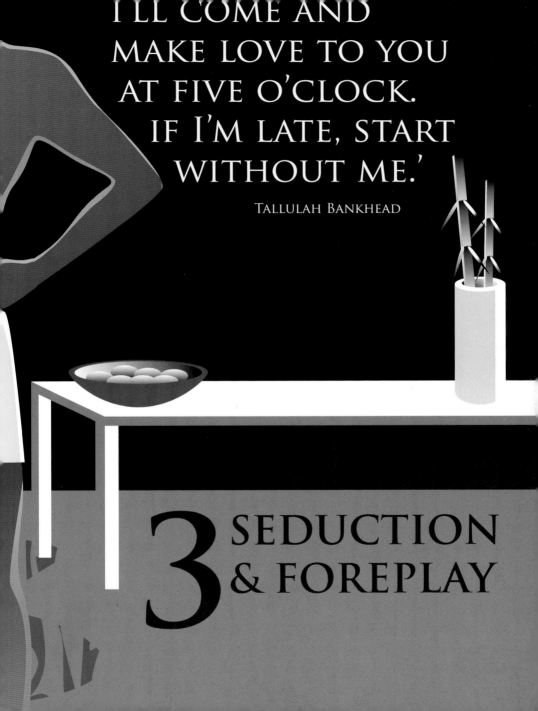

I'LL COME AND
MAKE LOVE TO YOU
AT FIVE O'CLOCK.
IF I'M LATE, START
WITHOUT ME.'

Tallulah Bankhead

3 SEDUCTION
& FOREPLAY

SEDUCTION & FOREPLAY

It can be difficult for anyone – even a sex goddess – to know when to transform heavy flirtation into actual seduction. It's often an awkward moment, when noses bump or zippers get stuck. As a trainee sex goddess you need to know how to move seamlessly from gazing into each other's eyes to slowly exploring each other's mouths, and then beyond. There comes a point, however, when it's easier to continue your lovemaking than to back off, clear your throat and offer to make a cup of tea. So if you decide you're going to go for it, it's helpful to pinpoint this 'Seduction Moment'.

You can, of course, wait for him to make the lip-locking first move. Sometimes it is just one look or moment between you and all else falls into place quite naturally. However, if he seems unsure as to whether you're really interested in him, you need to make it clear. A friend of mine simply leans forward and kisses the guy in mid-sentence – an effective but brave manoeuvre.

If that kind of action's too drastic for you, wait for him to pause for breath and then let your eyes deliberately drop to his mouth. You may even reach out and idly trail your hand down his arm, or stroke his fingers or even his face. If he fails to get the message after this, he may well be brain dead, in which case, what are you doing seducing him?

If you're prepared to give him a final chance, maintain your gaze on his lips while leaning very slightly forward – exactly the way it happens in movies when a couple is about to kiss and something dramatic prevents them at the last minute. Ideally, in your case nothing will, and you'll melt together painlessly. If he's shy, you'll need to do all of the above, but slower. If you are both shy, you will have to decide whether you would rather miss a golden opportunity than risk embarrassment. The truth is, it's not hard to tell if someone's interested. If they make all the right moves but pull back at the last minute, they're a champion game-player and you're better off without them.

'...from gazing into
each other's eyes
to slowly exploring
each other's mouths.'

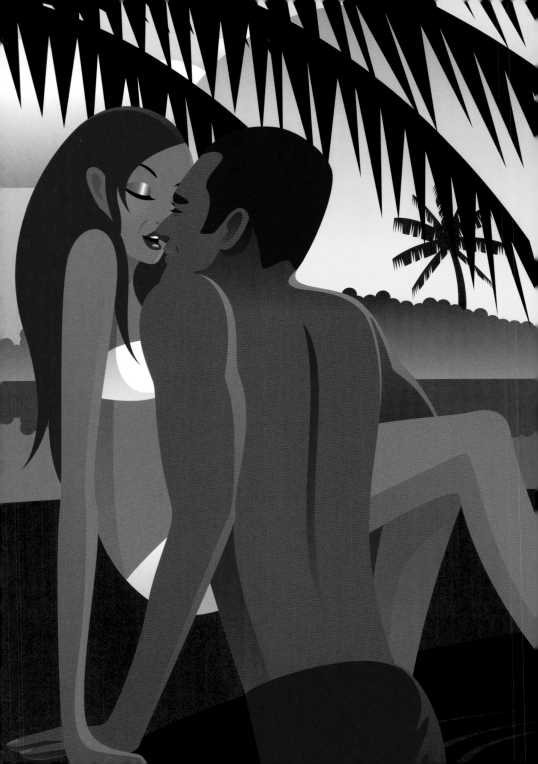

KISSING WITH CONFIDENCE

You might think everyone can kiss. But you'd be wrong. An alarming number of people assume that all they have to do is press their lips together and rotate their tongues for a bit. This is not, however, how a sex goddess kisses, and rightly so. A real kiss – the proper kind that makes him catch his breath to prevent him being overcome by erotic feelings and collapsing at your feet – requires a lot more than that.

The basic techniques is to begin with gentle pressure on the lips and gradually part them. A few more delicate presses on the sides of his mouth, then brush your lips up and down over his, by now, also parted, lips. There are thousands of nerve endings in the lips, and your aim should be to stimulate every one of them. All this comes before any tongue action. When you do introduce it, be subtle: no one wants their mouth forcefully invaded. Allow the tip of your tongue to dart out to meet his. Move it gently in an exploratory fashion – never let it lie in his mouth like a damp rag. Don't leave your tongue inside for too long though; keep breaking away and returning to lip kissing in order to build up the anticipation.

Sometimes you can move away from his mouth altogether and kiss his neck, just below his ear. For many people this is a major erogenous zone. Combine the kissing with a little stroking of his hair, neck or face, or body caressing, and… bang, you're off and running. If you're going to bite the neck area, though, be gentle. Most men won't appreciate a giant purple bruise blooming above their collars. Once you've mastered the art of sex-goddess kissing, you can move on to explore the rest of him.

KISSING TIPS

Kissing isn't as easy as it looks. There's an art to it, and clamping your mouths together and hoping for the best isn't it. A great kiss can be as good as sex, and sometimes better, because it's filled with promise as well as eroticism. So if you've never been quite sure you were doing it right, follow the advice below and you can't go wrong. And if his kiss isn't working for you, you might be able to improve it.

1. Let your lips brush together a couple of times before you home in. This builds tension and arouses all the nerve endings in your lips.

2. Always make sure your breath is divinely fresh. It sounds obvious, but after a night drinking and smoking, it's so going to smell like a bar floor. So nip off and eat a mint first, at least.

3. If he really can't kiss, the best way to retrain him is simply to say, 'Can I just tell you a little kissing trick that drives me wild with desire? Just keep still, and I'll show you.' Then proceed to kiss him exactly as you want to be kissed. It can't fail – all men want to drive women wild with desire.

4. Break off during the kiss to reposition your lips. This stimulates different nerves and makes sure the erotic charge keeps being released. There's nothing duller than a kiss where nobody moves.

5. Use your hands, too. Caress the back of his neck or run your fingers through his hair. Passionate clutching of his back is also a good move, as is sliding your hand inside his shirt or T-shirt, depending how far you really want the kiss to go, of course.

HOW TO TOUCH HIM

So long as you're not too heavy-handed or completely out of sync with each other, most sensory touching feels quite nice, but there's a world of difference between 'fairly pleasant', and 'Oh, my God'. Clearly, as a sex goddess you'll be aiming for the latter. Grasping a handful of the back of his sweater while wondering how you're going to get his jeans undone is not the best a man can get, believe me.

Sensual touch is a combination of tease and pressure. You want him to anticipate that you're heading for his erogenous zones, without actually touching them just yet, while at the same time, stimulating all his nerve endings so he's driven crazy with desire. A word about nipples. For most men, nipple touching is as personal as their taste in underwear and, without asking, it's almost impossible to guess what he wants. While some men adore a nipple-squeeze, a light pinch or a gently circling fingertip, others shudder in horror at the very idea. The only way to find out is to ask. You don't have to bring a halt to proceedings – a simple, murmured, 'Does that feel nice?' will suffice.

Arm stroking is a bit girly for many men, unlike most women, who love to be caressed all over with a fluttering touch. Men prefer any touching action to have a purpose. Basically, if they believe you're making them feel good shortly before heading straight down to their penis, they're happy. On the other hand, if they think you're engaged on some nebulous, tactile journey, they're likely to get bored and will attempt to push your hand downwards after a few minutes. While you're stroking and caressing him, keep reminding him of the ultimate goal: sweep one hand close to his genitals, even brush across them – and then prolong the teasing. That way, he'll be excited, not frustrated.

EROTIC MASSAGE

Experiment with touching by practising some massage strokes on your man, and hopefully he'll return the favour. The following instructions aren't exactly a massage, more of a prolonged exercise in the Art of Tease, and he will appreciate it as such.

1. Begin at his neck. Lightly stroke the base where it joins his collarbone and at the same time, gently squeeze the back of his neck to make him feel instantly relaxed, yet extremely turned on. The neck area is a very vulnerable part of the body and by caressing him here, you're creating a deeply intimate connection that's based on trust. Once you've gained his trust, you can do anything, right?

2. Now run your fingers down his spine, or slide your palms along it, rocking your hand slightly, to stimulate both sides of his back. Once you reach the base, lightly scratch your nails down his buttocks, before kneading them firmly.

3. Trail your hands along his inner and outer thighs and stroke the tops and soles of his feet with a firm sweep of your hand (otherwise it just feels ticklish and he'll probably either inadvertently kick you or giggle).

4. Now turn him over and touch his front; areas to concentrate on first include his hips, particularly the hollows just beneath them, and his stomach. It doesn't matter whether he has a washboard or a pillow, all stomachs respond well to gentle circling of the fingers, especially when you allow them to drift down towards his groin and teasingly pull back. Many men love to have their frequently neglected sides caressed, too, with light, sweeping motions up towards the chest.

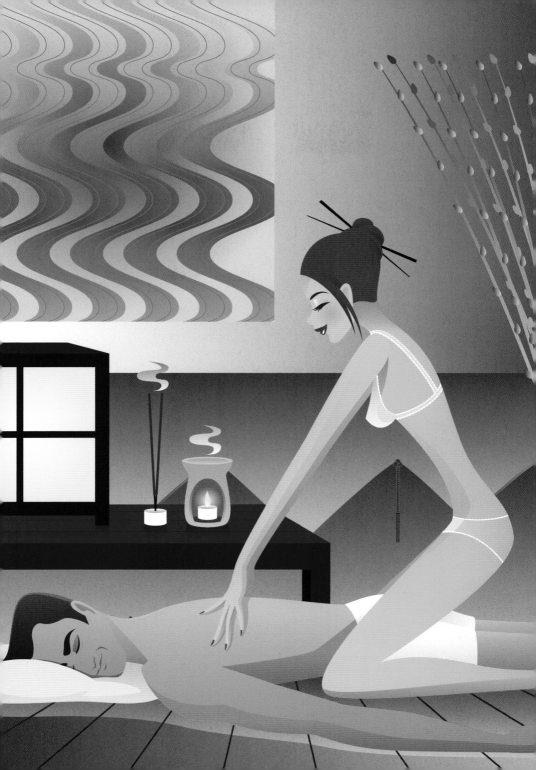

GETTING THE
RIGHT TOUCH FROM HIM

Obviously, you are a goddess of touch and he can't possibly complain about your technique. He, however, is not necessarily a god. When it comes to being touched, your challenge is to persuade him to do what you want without nagging or criticizing him, or making him think he's an inept fool with hands like hams. In the anxiety to please a new partner, some men may be a little awkward, so give him the benefit of the doubt first.

A lot of men are unsure when it comes to touching a woman. They've spent so long engaged in pleasing themselves (look, I'm sorry but it's true) that they naturally assume you want to be touched in the same way – firm, direct and straight to the genitals.

*'Your challenge
is to persuade
him to do what
you want.'*

Of course, women are more like artichokes. To please you he must nibble his way through lots of layers, which are enjoyable to toy with in their own right, before he gets right to the heart – your clitoris. There are two ways of teaching him this. The first, and most traditional one, is simply to guide his hands, to wriggle away in a coquettish manner every time he makes a beeline for your genitals and to make all the right noises when he does the right things, but stay quiet when things are less than exciting. Now this may work if he's the one man alive who understands exquisite subtlety, who grew up with five sisters and learned to decode the sighs and groans of women at twenty paces, and who also has a PhD in psychology. However, if he's a regular guy who didn't do these things, all you will end up with is him wondering why you're huffing and puffing and won't let him stroke you for two minutes without writhing around like a harpooned sandshark. So you might find the second, less traditional, teaching method works better. Read on…

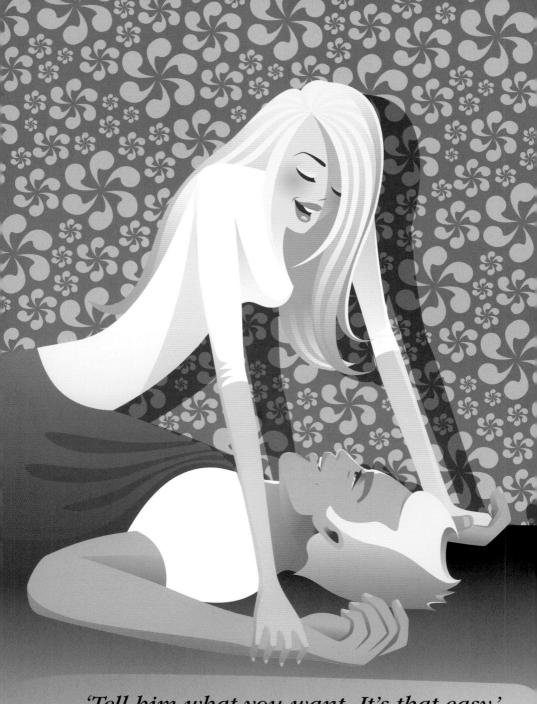

'Tell him what you want. It's that easy.'

BE UPFRONT

Tell him what you want. It's that easy. Like many women, you may now be clasping your hands like a coy Southern belle, murmuring, 'Oh, I couldn't. It's embarrassing. He'll think I'm demanding, he'll think he doesn't satisfy me…' Admittedly, it's hard to start laying down guidelines on the first night, though even then a simple 'Mmm, that feels amazing, just a bit to the right' shouldn't offend anyone. But if you intend to be with this man for more than 12 hours, do you really want to set up a pattern where he does it all wrong for you and you act like it's fine, a routine that could go on forever? Of course, a stream of barked instructions – 'OK, OK, touch me there. Harder. No, now. Rub me. Yes. No. You've slowed down, speed up.' – will make him feel more like a NASA mechanic than your lover and he may well send you spiralling into space accordingly. But there are subtler ways to tell him how to turn you on and any man worth making love to will be grateful for the information. A simple 'That feels wonderful, could you do it even a tiny bit faster?' is fine so long as you sound happy rather than irritable. Or 'I don't really come during sex, but if you could rub me afterwards that would be fantastic.' And if you're really lucky, 'Oh God. Please, hard as you can. You feel incredible.'

Use lots of positive adjectives and excitable tones. Compliment him and encourage him. Think of your man as a dog who's eager to please, but doesn't know if you want him to bring you the paper or your slippers. He needs kindly direction and lots of praise. It's better to do this in bed (or wherever you make love) than over dinner. Otherwise, you run the risk of it being more like an analyst's session: 'You know when you do that weird thing with your lips? What's going on there?' isn't nearly as sexy as, 'Oh, yes, don't stop' in the throes of passion.

Consider that what works for one woman may not be the same for another. He may have been in a long-term relationship and got used to pleasing one partner. You will need to make him feel at ease and appreciated, while gently leading him in the right direction.

HIS FAVOURITE THING

It is not exactly that it's all about his penis or anything… without it, he'd probably be just as happy going fishing or watching the sports on TV. Because for a man, a whole lot of sex really does come down to what his penis is feeling, which is why they're all so obsessed by size and judge their manliness accordingly. Therefore, it pays for you, a sex goddess in the making, to know exactly how to handle your man's penis. You'd think it would be easy, right? But you'd be amazed just how many women don't know how to manage a simple erection. For a start, some penises can look a bit purple and even threatening or perhaps a little off-putting. But if you think of his penis as his vulnerable alter ego, your attitude will be transformed. You will want to do right by him and, as we all know, you have to give a little to get a little.

You can add all sorts of fancy strokes to your basic handjob. The 'double hander', where you massage the base at the same time as the tip, is always enjoyable. Try the 'shaft massage', which is exactly as it says. Flex your fingers all the way up and back down. Or you can simply tease him by running your fingers around the head, while stroking the frenulum – the tiny bit of skin joining the head and shaft – with your thumb.

'Think of his penis as his vulnerable alter ego, your attitude will be transformed.'

Once you've got the basic method down, the rest should come easily, as it were. When he starts to come, the most sex-goddess thing you can do is to lean down and swallow his semen. If that's about as appealing as eating a bucket of slugs (really, it's not that bad, but some girls are terribly fastidious), the second best thing is to allow him to come all over your breasts. This is always a good one combined with the penis-rubbing-between-the-breasts technique. Failing that, let him ejaculate on your butt or, if he's after a dirty porn-type experience, your face.

But if you're not feeling that generous, there's always your stomach. What, still a no? Then point his penis towards his stomach. The bonus to this option is that the sheets won't get messed up. Have some tissues handy by the bed, too, as there's nothing quite so odd as the feeling of sperm drying on the skin.

And when it comes to him touching your clitoris the right way, make sure he returns the compliment. Tell him exactly what you want him to do – he'll love it, and so will you.

HANDLE WITH CARE

Most men prefer a firm grip on their penis. Unfortunately, many women make the fundamental error – just as some men can do with women – of handling a penis in the same way they'd enjoy having their clitoris fondled: gently and delicately. But his favourite thing is far more robust than that. He needs to be held confidently, or you won't get the necessary rhythm going, and the friction will be lacklustre to say the least.

1

So grasp his penis
in your right (or left) hand
as if you're holding onto a glass
and don't want it to slip – obviously
you're not squeezing so hard it will
break, either. Your little finger should
be at the base and your thumb round
the top. That leaves your other hand
free for fondling balls, nipples,
anus, thighs, and so on,
as desired.

'Most men prefer a firm grip on their penis.'

2

Once you've got the grip right (don't worry, he'll let you know – he's had years of practice), you can begin to move your hand up and down. The skin of his penis should move but your fingers shouldn't shift at all – the action is all in the wrist. If he's circumcised or has a tight foreskin that won't move back and forth easily, you may need to move your fingers. Lubrication – a pea-sized amount as it says on the tube – should do the job.

3

Build up your speed gradually until you're rubbing as fast as you can stand without hurting your wrist. However, always keep the rhythm steady – no sudden pulls or jerks, and no grinding to a halt just as he's beginning to gasp.

ORAL SEX

Possibly one of the greatest inventions known to man, and woman, is oral sex. It can, however, be fraught with difficulty, because women are so often nervous of receiving it and wary of giving it. We worry about how we look, taste and smell. We fret that he might be bored and when it comes to giving blow jobs, we're too often torn between fear of getting it wrong and the pain of a numb jaw. There are ways to make oral sex nothing but enjoyable – and they're very simple.

HOW TO RECEIVE IT

Having him go down on you is a lovely display of trust and passion. If he's down there, it's because he wants to be, so don't ruin it by muttering, 'Oh no, God, I haven't washed for at least an hour.' If you're that worried, wash just before you come to bed, and rest assured that men are programmed to find the smell and taste of a healthy vagina perfectly erotic.

If he isn't doing what you like with his tongue there is a relatively foolproof method that virtually guarantees oral orgasm, which you can teach him. To begin, he should part your labia gently with his thumb and forefinger; then locate your clitoris with his tongue. But instead of licking all over it randomly, he should simply flick his tongue back and forth across the 'hood' of the clitoris and round the edges, where sensitivity is at its height. If he also pushes a finger slowly in and out of your vagina at the same time, you should soon be coming round the mountain, in no uncertain terms.

Remember that if he's bothering to do this, it's because he wants to please you – so show him exactly what you want and don't just lie there wishing he'd get it over with as he frantically nibbles the wrong spot. Sometimes men are too rough, allow their teeth to nip you or even imagine that violent sucking is a good idea. In which case, tell him it isn't. His next girlfriend will thank you for it.

HOW TO GIVE IT

Giving a blowjob is not always a simple case of 'you just put your lips together and suck'. While that will keep him happy for quite some time, there are more sophisticated techniques that will ensure you're both enjoying yourselves.

One of the most important considerations is your position. Lying down with your head between his legs will last about two minutes until it starts to hurt. The best ways to give a comfortable blow job are: one, lying at right angles to his body, with your head sideways on his lap; and two, kneeling between his legs while he sits upright. The first way works because you can angle his penis to bump against your cheek, not your tonsils, which removes all risk of gagging. If it still feels too big, flex your jaw and he'll pop further out whether he wants to or not.

You can supplement your mouth with your hand around the base, and rub in rhythm with your head movements. Start off reasonably slowly, with your lips closed around the head of his penis, just taking the shaft into your mouth and out a little way. As he gets more excited you can speed up. By using your hand, you can save yourself the exhaustion of bobbing your head frantically. Because your mouth's a bit freer this way, you can also use your tongue to stroke and caress the tip or to flick along the shaft. You can supplement the basic blow job technique with a mouthful or warm liquid, or champagne, which feels incredible swirled around his sensitive parts. But make sure you keep your lips clamped shut, and your teeth firmly out of the way. You can also pay his balls attention – licking, sucking and gentle fondling will all feel marvellous, but nibbling, pulling and squeezing will not. You can try 69, which involves you simultaneously going down on each other, but it can be difficult to focus on what you're feeling and what you're doing at the same time: it is a good party trick if you can manage it.

'The big question, of course, is Spit or Swallow?'

The big question, of course, is Spit or Swallow? It's entirely up to you, but swallowing is very generous and very sexy. Just let it all hit the back of your throat, hold it in your mouth and keep your tongue still if you don't want to taste it. Then gulp. And you can always have a drink straight afterwards. If you spit, be discreet – it's only kind, after all.

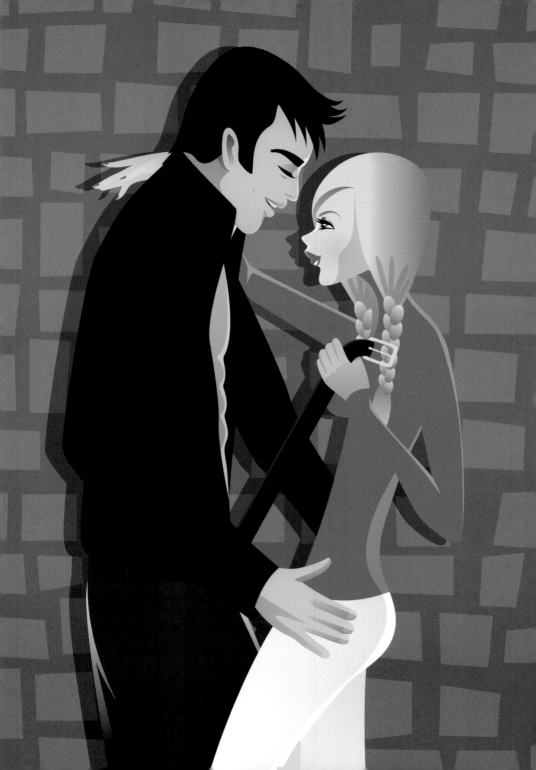

TOP FIVE FOREPLAY TIPS

1

A massage may sound a bit dull and worthy, but for the stressed goddess, it's an invaluable way to get in the mood for sex. Explain to him that if he devotes 20 minutes to kneading and stroking you, you'll devote 20 minutes to licking and sucking him, and you should have a bargain.

2

If you're struggling to get yourself in the mood, focus on a very sexual memory, and recall how you felt and what you could hear, see, smell and taste. This way, you can reconnect with how it felt to be deeply sexually involved, and your brain will trigger the same chemicals and endorphins.

'...if he devotes 20 minutes to kneading and stroking you, ...you'll devote 20 minutes to licking and sucking him.'

3

Don't ignore the area between his balls and bottom – called the perineum. It responds remarkably well to light pressure, or small circles of your fingertip. Don't press too hard, but if you combine it with a handjob, he'll be your slave forever. Probably.

4

Teach him to kiss your neck and ears as well as your breasts. Many men have a habit of going straight for the obvious body parts, but most women have deeply erogenous zones around the sides of the neck and just below the ears. Light kissing or licking around these areas can be almost as good as an orgasm, and certainly make you want one pretty fast.

5

Most women need to be seduced relatively slowly. So if he makes a habit of grabbing your nipples and expecting instant delight, you must remind him that, generally, kissing comes first. It brings you closer emotionally, it's deeply intimate and you'll be much more inclined to get your nipples out afterwards. If you can't remember the last time you had a good snog, there's something very wrong, but it can easily be sorted out.

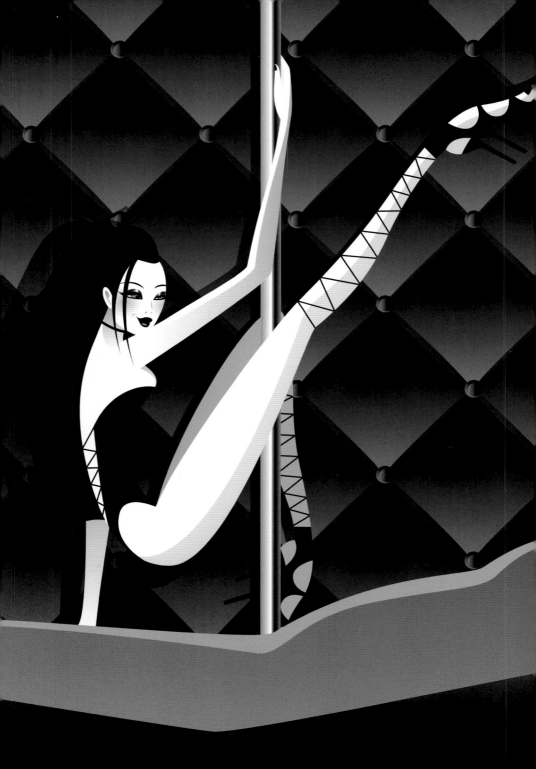

'THERE ARE NO GOOD GIRLS GONE WRONG, JUST BAD GIRLS FOUND OUT.'

MAE WEST

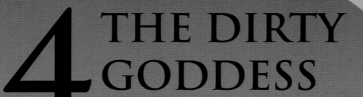

4 THE DIRTY GODDESS

WHAT TO WEAR IN BED

It's easier to tell you what not to wear first. Avoid anything featuring cartoon characters, cute slogans like 'Cuddle Me' or 'I Need A Hug' ('I Need a Sick Bag', more like) or anything made of brushed cotton. Unless he has a granny fetish, it's unlikely he'll be tempted to find out what's underneath your floral-sprigged, tent-size nightie. Boudoir wear is an art. If you're planning to be a sex goddess, it's not acceptable to throw on a ripped, oversized old T-shirt every night. Comfortable though it is, it's not a look that screams 'Take me'.

Listen carefully, aspiring sex goddesses. There's a world of difference between 'dirty goddess' and 'dirty slut'. Dirty sluts have no self-respect and will let a man do whatever he wants, however degrading. Dirty goddesses, however, enjoy the raunch potential of sex. They know that good sex isn't all about candlelight, soft music and gentle caresses. Sometimes only hard, filthy fucking will do. But that kind of sex doesn't mean your partner won't respect you, or that you have to degrade yourself. So long as you want to do it, and you're equally turned on, you can be as 'dirty' as you like without any worries. And if you're not happy with something, you tell him so. You don't say, 'OK, I'll do it with all your friends from the bar so you like me more'. Because dirty goddess sex is only as dirty as you want it to be.

Your partner may feel that you are taking him for granted and failing to make an effort. Of course, lots of women – and men – like to sleep naked. There's no harm in that and it certainly encourages bodily contact, but it's a little like serving the dessert before you've had the appetizer – it kind of ruins the surprise. Men's sexuality is based largely on anticipation, so for him it's far more exciting to present yourself as a delightful present ready to be slowly unwrapped rather than as a wholesome Swedish type who's about to go hiking au naturel. Most likely, he

'...sometimes only hard,
filthy fucking will do.'

will make the final decision on what he wants to wear in bed, and sadly the options for sexy male bedroom-wear are limited. A fresh pair of underpants to show off his shape will probably work for you. If you're choosing a seduction outfit for him, bear in mind that cotton, silk or nothing at all suits all men and, as with your own bed-wear, avoid any with cartoons or slogans. I hardly need to mention that posing pouches are about as sexy as paunches, do I? Thought not.

Despite the variety of gorgeous lingerie shops, some men are still really bad at buying sex-wear for women. Crotchless scarlet lace rarely enhances anybody's best bits, unless their labia happen to be particularly stunning. If he's buying, head him in the direction of one of the many lingerie emporiums offering edgy, sexy but well-made items. Rather than nylon nasties you'll be getting something that will feel great against your skin and put you in the mood. Convince him that this is something that will ultimately benefit him. And as for sleeping, there are plenty of sexy nightdresses that won't compromise on comfort or style – train your eyes to slide past anything featuring cartoon sheep. Although sex-wear is not the same thing as sleepwear, the two can be combined in the form of, say, a see-through baby-doll. However, do keep a selection of 'boudoir-wear' aside for special romantic occasions; there'll be no doubt as to what's on the agenda if he sees you in this. Your sex-wear should consist of at least one outfit (or single item) that enhances all your assets and makes you feel devastatingly sexy.

When buying underwear, don't worry about whether the items will show underclothes. Instead ask yourself, 'Do I look a million dollars in this?' Look for lace (though not the scarlet scratchy kind), silk, satin, ribbons, mesh and bows. Cleavage-enhancing corsetry or tight-fitting but silky gowns will show off your figure. Most men are wildly excited by red or purple underwear, so consider deviating from basic black. Obviously avoid stretch nylon, sporty cotton and anything serviceable that looks as though you could carry shopping home in it. Pretty G-strings are great, small panties fine, but big, sensible butt-grippers are not. The best ones are those that tie at the sides – sometimes known as 'stripper-knickers'.

Admittedly, some men like white, virginal underwear. But if you're unsure, go for the 'classy whore' look – it'll get you everywhere. Make sure your bra is professionally fitted – four breasts are not a good look. Hate your stomach? Buy a vintage-style, wide, lacy suspender (garter) belt to give you an air of 1950s glamour, or choose a basque or a corset, to which you can attach stockings.

Ah yes, hosiery… There are some men who actually prefer tights (pantyhose), but they tend to have grown up in the 1970s when 'American Tan' was not yet a term of abuse. On the whole, you're safer with stockings. Go for black, barely black or fishnet. Unless you are very thin or getting married, avoid white hosiery, they'll make your legs look like undercooked sausages.

For guaranteed sex appeal you are much safer with stockings or lacy hold-ups. They look great, provide easy access to underwear (which always goes on top of suspenders (garters), never underneath), and they tap directly into every man's sexual fantasy list. Generally, suspenders are sexier than hold-ups because they are more traditional and don't leave strange, pink elastic-marks round your thighs. If they're just too fiddly to put on, leave the hold-ups on throughout sex and he'll be so excited, he'll never know the difference.

ACCESSORIES AND FOOT FETISHES

Naturally, most women wouldn't normally wear shoes to bed. But even if you're a sporty sneaker-girl who walks like a newborn giraffe in high heels, a pair of 'boudoir shoes' is a good investment. 'Lay-me-down-and-fuck-me' shoes (as they are technically known) feature stiletto heels, ankle straps or ribbons and pointy toes. They have the effect of elongating your legs and enhancing the curve of your butt – and also putting your man in mind of a little light bondage. Obviously feminism is not making its presence overtly clear here, but you can always lecture him later on equal rights once you've tied him to the bedpost.

Of course, the old 'hooker' standby of thigh-high boots is also a winner in the bedroom – but only if you've got legs like Julia Roberts in *Pretty Woman*, otherwise you run the risk of looking like *Puss in Boots*. Much safer are marabou fluffy mules, as worn by Marilyn Monroe and a variety of 1950s glamour models. Supplement your boudoir range with a selection of négligés, silk wraps, peignoirs and kimonos to float around the house. Add chiffon shawls, long strings of pearls, and even chain belts and diamond piercings – fake ones if you don't fancy suffering unnecessary pain just to draw attention to your erogenous zones.

Of course, everyone knows how to undress, but not everyone can undress like a sex goddess. When it comes to sex, just pulling off your clothes and throwing them in a heap won't do, unless you both fancy a quickie. There are two types of undressing, sex goddess style: Sexy Disrobing and Actual Stripping.

SEXY DISROBING

The natural moment for a little sexy disrobing is when you're getting ready for bed or changing clothes. Even if you don't have access to a thumping backing track or the energy to slink around in front of him wearing a feather boa for 10 minutes, you can still offer him a treat.

Avoid taking your shoes off at first – you'll immediately look much shorter and, therefore, less sexy. However this rule does not apply if you're wearing sports shoes or hiking boots, so get 'em off. Remember, always leave the best until last, so next slowly remove your jeans or skirt, giving him a great view of your legs as you undo your top.

There's no harm in turning away and bending down as you do this, though you must keep your legs straight or it's no use at all as an erotic pose. Once you're down to your bra and knickers (panties), you can offer him the chance to undo your bra for you, or just whip it off. Now bend down (straight legs, remember) and slowly ease down your panties.

Even skimpy G-strings or tricky suspender (garter) belts can be removed elegantly if you keep your legs straight, and once your underwear is off you could even fling the item at him playfully. Straighten up and turn to face him, delightfully naked.

You may like to remove your shoes at this point. If you're wearing tights (pantyhose), discount the shoe advice and remove these first – otherwise you'll look like an extra in a Jane Fonda workout video. Besides, tights make it almost impossible for him to touch you or to gain access to your body, and they definitely look better under clothes than they do on their own. This method of stripping off is the simplest way to get undressed and still keep his rapt attention.

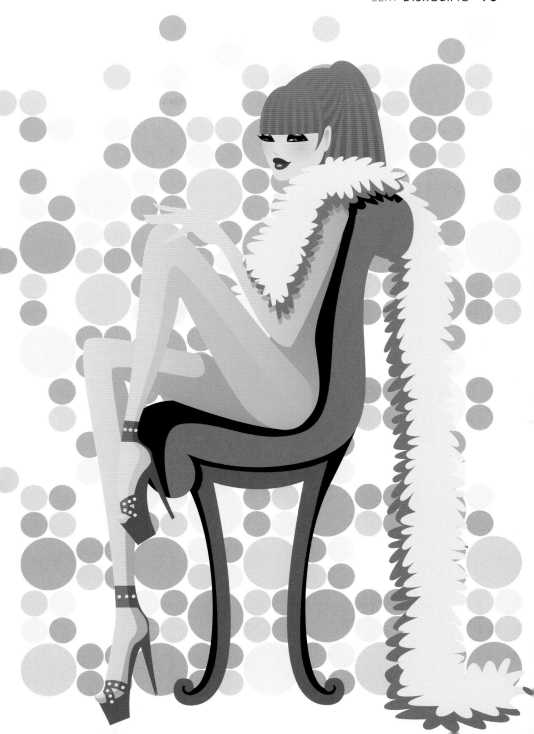

TOP TEN STEPS TO SUCCESSFUL STRIPPING

1. Place your hands on the fastening of your top and stroke your fingers over the zipper or buttons to give the impression that you might just possibly be thinking about undoing them.

2. Maintaining seductive eye contact, slide the zipper down or undo the buttons, and then turn away from him and remove your top. Keeping your hands over your breasts, turn back to face him.

3. Slide your hands down over your hips to your skirt fastening. Again, play with the zipper – slide it down a little one way then back up again to tease him.

4. Undo your skirt or trousers and turn away again. Now bend forward a little (straight legs, naturally) and allow your clothes to fall to the floor. If it's a small garment, kick it aside or use the toe of your shoe to toss it upwards, catch it and fling it to him.

5. With your hands over your breasts, face him again and dance slowly, gliding your hands up and down your body. Slide a bra strap down and then back up to tease him. Let both straps drop but keep your bra in place with your hands. Reach down to the back and unclip it, but don't let it drop yet…

6. Now turn away again so he can admire your butt. Let your bra fall, and then reach down gracefully and throw it to him while still facing away from him. Place your hands over your breasts and turn back to face him. To reveal your breasts, slowly slide your hands down to the sides of your knickers (panties). (You did remember to put your knickers on *over* the suspenders, didn't you?)

7. Tease him a bit more. Pull the sides of your knickers down a little way, or pretend to undo the ribbons. Push the front down as far as it will go without revealing any pubic hair. Turn round again and slip your knickers down then step out of them neatly. Kick them aside, or to him.

8. Nearly there. Except for shoes and stockings, you are now naked and it's perfectly acceptable to stop at this point if you want. But if you prefer full nudity, take off your shoes. Standing on one leg, undo each clip. (If you're less flexible, place one foot at a time on the bed, or rest your foot on the chair he's sitting on and slowly roll each stocking down, then pull it off with a flick of the wrist.) Reach down to unclip your suspender (garter) belt and whip it away.

9. Continue to dance in front of him just out of reach until he can't bear it another second. You may then cross the room and begin to undress him.

10. If you're shy, and most of us are when it comes to taking off our clothes in a lit room, conceal as you reveal with a strategically placed feather boa. You can also add glamorous old-school accessories such as elbow-length gloves, a string of beads or a silk scarf. Use them to add to your performance, covering yourself with the boa or scarf as you slowly remove your lingerie.

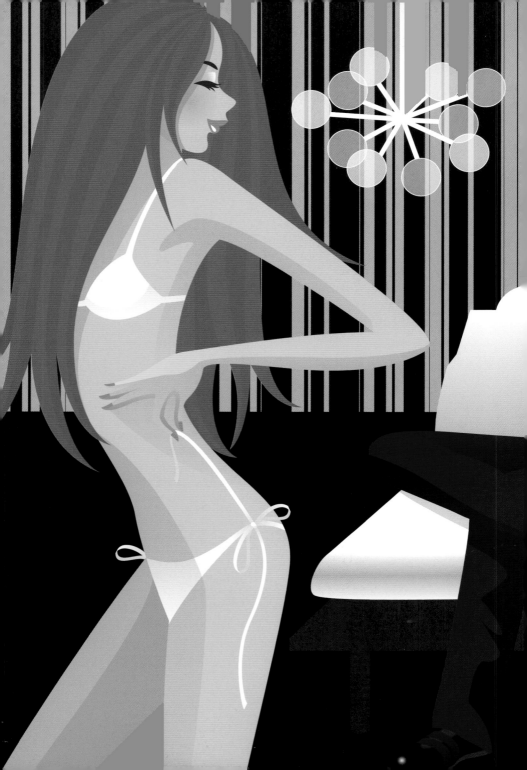

THE FULL STRIP

This is a more complex but ultimately satisfying method of disrobing. Of course you'll need music to do this, otherwise you'll just resemble a character in some weird art house film. Your audience (I'm assuming it's just one, but don't let me stop you) should be seated at a safe distance away from you so there will be no touching. The whole point of the striptease is to build sexual tension, so make sure you move close to him as you dance, and then writhe away frustratingly at the last minute.

Your backing track should have a good thumping, dirty beat – R&B goes down well – and make sure it's slow enough for you to remove your clothes in a leisurely fashion to avoid flinging everything off randomly in a desperate bid to keep up with the tune. The whole experience should be relaxed and sensuous for you both.

Wear clothes that are easy to remove, such as slippery satin. Avoid fiddly buttons, trousers and anything you have to squeeze over your head – hurricane hair is not a sexy look. A dress that does up at the front is ideal, or a front-fastening top and a split skirt. Underneath, wear stockings or hold-ups, knickers (panties), a bra or basque and, of course, the ubiquitous high heels so beloved of all men. Once you are dressed, the music is ready and you have some props to hand, you can follow the Top Ten Steps to Successful Stripping on pages 74–75.

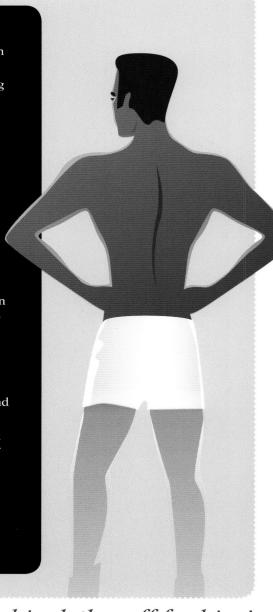

MALE STRIPPING

While there may be some women out there who get immensely turned on at the idea of watching a man strip, I don't know many of them. Women are less visually aroused than men at the sight of a naked body of the opposite sex, possibly because, unless they're having sex or taking a shower, naked men tend to look slightly ridiculous, even a little vulnerable. But if it floats your boat to watch him prancing around to 'Rock Your Body' in white socks and a posing pouch, go girl. If not, then come join the rest of us and take his clothes off for him.

Start by slowly unbuttoning his shirt, then slide it off. Run your fingers around his belt buckle and undo it. Unzip his trousers, put your hands on his hips and push so his jeans and boxers come off together. This only works if he's not wearing shoes; so if he is, help him to take them off first.

'...take his clothes off for him.'

TALKING DIRTY

To be a true sex goddess you need to cover all the senses. Looking good and smelling sweet – even having silken skin that tastes of rose petals – is not enough on its own. You've got to talk it like you walk it; in other words, you need to learn to talk dirty. Of course you can have silent, passionate sex, the only sound being the rustle of sheets and maybe the creak of kneejoints. It can be quite exciting to stifle your orgasm at times; for example when you're staying with family or having sex somewhere you shouldn't. But sometimes you need to voice your thoughts out loud if you want your true desires to be fulfilled – and most men are as responsive to this as a cat to the sound of a tin opener.

Goddess or not, the trouble is that dirty talk doesn't come naturally to most of us. For a start, 'dirty' words are generally the ones we've been taught as nice little girls never, ever to use. Overcoming the vision of your mother gasping in horror and disgust can be tough enough for some, and then there's the question of how to make your string of smut sound raunchy and convincing enough and not like an 11-year-old trying to impress her mates.

Rather than waiting until you're mid-sex, and then blurting out, 'Fuck me harder with your… er, um, your… well, OK, your rod' it pays to have a vague plan regarding the sort of things you can say that will turn both of you on. On the whole, men are aroused by earthy sexual language and like you to be direct. It won't do you any good if you meander on about him putting his jade stalk into your scarlet love box – he may well assume you've begun collecting Chinese artefacts and might wonder why you're bringing it up just now, mid-thrust.

Most men like plain, straightforward words, words that do what they say on the label, such as 'Cum', 'Fuck' and 'Cunt'. If just reading this is making you cringe, you may need a little practice. Some women find the word 'cunt' offensive, though they are quite happy using male-oriented sex slang. Of course what you say needs to turn you on as well, so if talking like a fourth-century warlord on a pillaging spree fails to drive you crazy with desire, a compromise can be reached.

BUILDING YOUR SEX LEXICON

If you're a shy goddess, the best way to begin to talk dirty is to establish the kind of things you'd like to say to your partner. Sit down with your man and both write down twenty words or phrases that turn you on. For inspiration, look at published erotica, think of scenes from your favourite movies or simply rummage through the dark closets of your sexual psyches. When you've finished, take turns to read out a phrase each – yours might be 'I love your beautiful body', while his could be the more direct, 'I want to fill you with my hot cum'. Either way, you'll soon find out what excites your partner. Then swap and read out each other's lists. Vary your speed and tone, put on a French or Italian accent and have fun. The idea is to get used to speaking the words out loud. He may have no problem saying the word 'fuck', but really struggle with 'love'. You might find 'gorgeous' really easy, but clam up over 'cock'. It's like learning a foreign language, so practise until you both feel comfortable and you can start putting words together.

'...get used to speaking the words out loud.'

TALKING IN BED TOGETHER

So you've learned to talk dirty while fully clothed and at the kitchen table, giggling like school kids. The hard part (see how easily it slips out?) is to do this in the throes of passion. Begin during foreplay so you get used to the sound of each other's voices. Describe how you're feeling – a simple 'God, that's fantastic!' will suffice. As the action heats up, so will your words and hopefully, before you know it, you'll be giving each other an erotic running commentary. Bear in mind, though, that unless it's used sparingly, talking dirty can soon turn into a tedious monologue. You don't want to be begging for his hot tool only to find he's gone to look for his earplugs.

THE SEX GODDESS AND PORN

Porn can be a fraught subject. Most women don't enjoy the thought of their partners flicking through a magazine full of 17-year-olds with breasts bigger than their IQs, or the idea of him masturbating over some inflatable on-screen stunner. It can make us feel insecure and jealous and that's not to mention any stronger feelings we may harbour about the role of porn and its often-misogynist image.

If you hate porn, fair enough – I won't suggest you get over it and learn to love the sight of eight jiggling boobs and one squashed-looking guy, who's supposed to encapsulate all our fantasies. While most porn is still aimed at men, the good news is that sections of the industry are finally waking up to the notion that women might want to watch something that turns them on, too. Ex-porn actress Candida Royale has produced a series of female-friendly videos and others are following. Internet retailers mean that there's no need to shuffle round sex shops to choose a film. Watching porn together works well for some couples, though plenty of women find they'd rather not, due to potential insecurity. There's also the danger they may forget about sex completely and end up shrieking with laughter, saying, 'What is that hair about?' or 'Is that 1985 or what?' instead. If you do want to go for it, allow your own action to develop alongside whatever's going on on-screen. Sitting side by side, watching in silence, is a little too much like frequenting a sleazy sex cinema – unless of course that idea turns you on. And if 'blue movie' action doesn't work, you could always try some shared viewing of internet sites or looking at magazines together.

'...allow your own action to develop alongside whatever's going on on-screen.'

ALL IN THE MIND

If none of the above appeals, then try women's porn (aka erotic literature). Some years ago, publishing houses realized that many women enjoy reading about sex, more than watching it. Hence the sudden flood of erotica with blurry black-and-white photos of orgasmic women on the front covers, breathlessly titled *The Blue Pearl* or *The Taming of Theresa*, and so on. The stories generally focus on heroines who somehow keep stumbling upon cruel, hard masters and their wayward bisexual mistresses, but hey, it's more fun than reading cookbooks in bed. If the florid writing style leaves you cold, try more mainstream literature with an erotic bent, by writers such as Anaïs Nin, Colette, the Marquis de Sade (why are they all French, I wonder?), Nancy Friday, Vladimir Nabokov or Henry Miller, or classics such as *Moll Flanders, Lady Chatterley's Lover* or *Fanny Hill*. Read them out loud to each other or steal away somewhere and get yourself all worked up alone. (If you decide to read them in the bath, don't drop the book in your excitement – they're hell to dryout.)

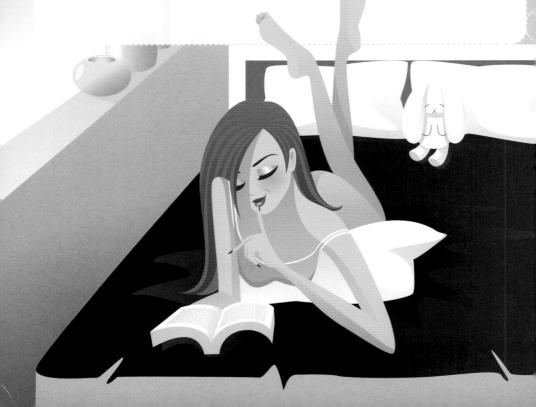

TOP FIVE PORN TIPS FOR DIRTY GODDESSES

1. *Nerve* magazine at www.nerve.com provides a wealth of couple-friendly erotica. There are stories, confessionals and a library of erotic photos from the early days of photography ('Hold this fern and look winsome, Alicia') to more recent styles ('Cup your boob job, Shannon'). Either way, it works.

2. Cliterati at www.cliterati.co.uk is a fantasy site where women post their own sexual fantasies. Some are appallingly written, others merely dull, while still more… well, it's nice to know others are having the same thoughts. The site is helpfully divided into 'Straight', 'Gay', 'Taboo' and so on.

3. Nancy Friday is perhaps the pioneer of sexual openness. She produced a series of fantastic books on women's (and one on men's) sexual fantasies. *My Secret Garden, Forbidden Flowers, Women on Top* and *Men in Love* are jam-packed with things you may never have considered fantasizing about before, but now you mention it…

4. Join an organization or go to events that promote women's sexuality: Cake, operating in both the USA and UK, is dedicated to promoting women's sexuality in a positive light (more fun than it sounds) and regularly hosts huge parties with male and female lap dancers, party-goers in skimpy costumes and exotic dancers. No men are allowed in without a woman so it's a safe, fun place to drop your inhibitions. For more information, contact www.cakenyc.com.

5 *The Lover's Guide*: This ever-popular video series features real couples making love in an entertaining and instructive fashion. It's mainly entertaining, though, and it's 'porn' for people who object to the fakeness of most erotic film-making. This is the real thing with the loving aspect included. It's stylishly lit, decently scripted and very female friendly.

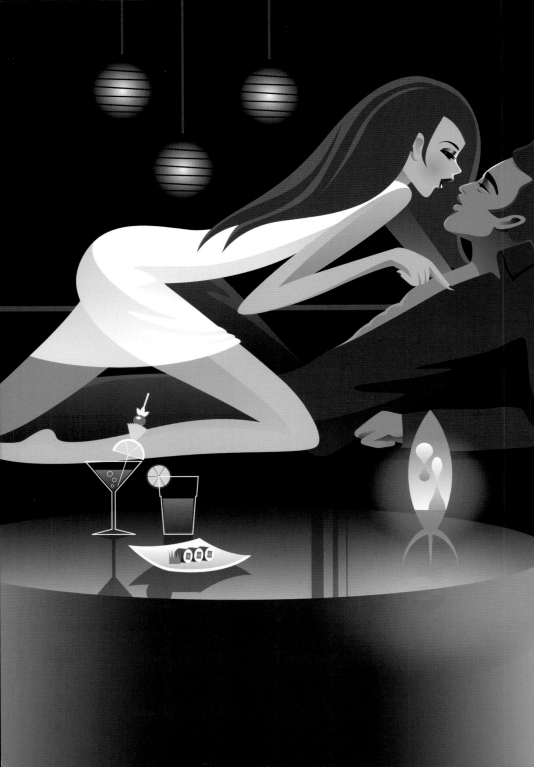

'I THINK PEOPLE SHOULD BE FREE TO ENGAGE IN ANY SEXUAL PRACTICES THEY CHOOSE; THEY SHOULD DRAW THE LINE AT GOATS, THOUGH.'

ELTON JOHN

5 XXX SEX & HOW TO HAVE IT

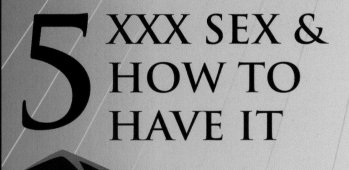

If you read magazines regularly (or even, like me, write for them regularly), you'd be forgiven for thinking that Actual Sex is the easiest thing in the world to get right. 'Your Best Sex Ever!', 'Make Mine A Large One – Multiple Orgasms!', 'Keep On Coming!': all these headlines are guaranteed to depress and trouble almost anybody. Because we're not all having this mythical Great Sex, we naturally assume there's something wrong with us – or else we're doing it wrong. Well, that may be true, but the genuine goddess knows that intercourse is not the be-all and end-all, and that great sex, as we've discussed already, is as much about attitude as it is about action.

That said, intercourse is still pretty important and there are various ways to make it work better for both parties. If you're not in the mood, your bodies don't fit together brilliantly or you expect a multiple orgasm after three thrusts, you probably will not have your Best Sex Ever. So the number-one tip for all sex goddesses is 'Have realistic expectations'.

'...great sex, is as much about attitude as it is about action.'

GREAT EXPECTATIONS

When having sex for the first time, both of you are going to be nervous – unless you're hopelessly drunk, in which case the chances are you won't be having great sex anyway. So expecting all that hanging-from-the-ceiling, screaming-with-joy stuff is almost certainly going to leave you disappointed by the average performances you'll both turn in.

But good sex isn't about any preconceived notions gleaned from glossy magazines or great cinematic moments, it's about – repeat after me – confidence and communication. Both build up over time, so first-night sex, particularly if you care about him, isn't going to be as good as third-month sex, when you can discuss what you want with ease. And if you're not emotionally involved, it can still be fantastic. As Woody Allen once said, 'Sex without love is an empty experience – but as empty experiences go, it's one of the best.' Don't beat yourself up over sex. If it's not perfect, read on, and you'll have all the technical knowledge at your fingertips. What only you can work out, however, is whether or not the guy's worth having sex with. So, even if you follow all the advice in the world, if the sex is still no good, it may be down to your choice of partner.

Anyone who's ever flicked through the Kama Sutra will know that there are at least 200 positions for sex. Anyone who's ever learned to drive a car, however, will know that it's complicated enough to get the gears and clutch working in harmony. Like driving, sex works best when it's smooth and simple. Don't expect to memorize hundreds of positions. It's enough to establish a repertoire of about ten, which work every time and deliver satisfaction all round. And the following are ten of the best…

THE MISSIONARY

This position is still the most popular, so it can't be bad. Missionary may be a little dull, but lying flat on your back, with him on top, gives you plenty of opportunities to kiss, knead his bottom and thrust your hips. You can liven it up by grinding them in circles, or press your thighs together instead of opening your legs so he feels as though he's penetrating a double-length vagina. You're clenching his penis between your thighs, even when he pulls out to thrust back into you. This also increases friction for you so it's a winner all round.

'…you're clenching his penis between your thighs.'

GIRL ON TOP

Favoured by women who like to be in control, this position works particularly well if he's got a large penis because you get to control the speed and depth of his thrusting. Insecurity is the enemy of girl-on-top ('Do my breasts look droopy?' 'Is he looking at my stomach?'). In fact, facing him from above, with your back arched so your breasts are thrust towards him is one of the most flattering positions you can get into. It also means you can lean forward so that your clitoris grinds against his pelvic bone, and the chances of an orgasm during sex are vastly enhanced. As a bonus, he doesn't have to use his hands for supporting his body so he is free to touch you.

SQUAT POSITION

A variation of girl-on-top, the squat isn't dignified, but it is orgasmic. Again, you're on top but instead of sitting down, you squat over him. Yes, it's a little like the position you'd adopt for peeing at a rock festival, but the rewards are infinitely greater. Wear high heels because your thighs will ache less. Gradually lower yourself onto his penis and lever yourself up and down by pressing your hands against his chest. This position stimulates your entire vagina, including your G-spot (if, indeed, you have one), and allows him to touch your clitoris and breasts so it's probably the best of all positions for any sex goddess – just so long as you have strong thighs.

'Wear high heels.'

OFF THE BED

Remember Jessica Lange and Jack Nicholson in *The Postman Always Rings Twice*? Well, even if you don't, the sexual position they made famous is an Oscar winner. She was on her back (on a flour-covered kitchen table as it happens, but it's just as good on a bed) and he stood between her legs. This means your man can achieve a powerful level of thrusting, either by holding onto the bed/table, or by gripping your hips. You can also raise your legs and balance your ankles on his shoulders to allow him maximum access to your vagina, and thus increase the friction. This is a passionate, male-dominant pose, plus it's one that works well half-clothed. So it's perfect if you're in a rush, like Jessica and Jack.

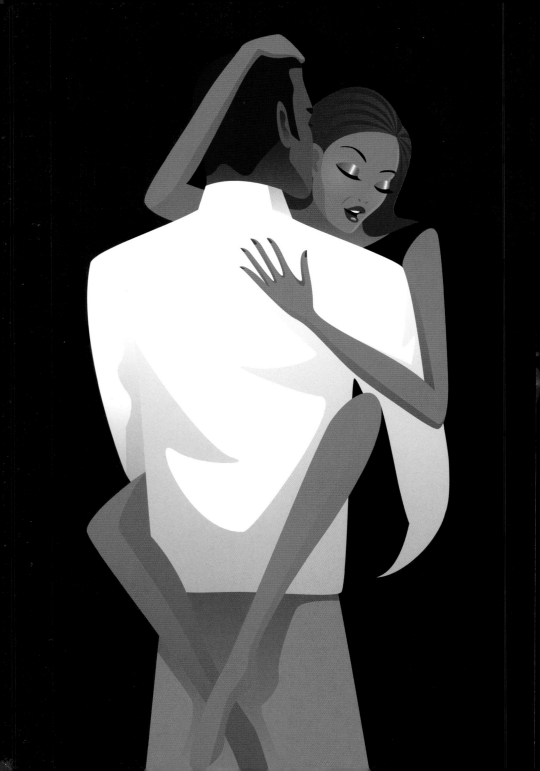

STANDING UP

Standing-up sex is much maligned because most people don't understand the basic principle. They think you have to be the same height, or that she has to fasten her legs round his waist like some tentacular giant squid. But the only standing-up sex that really works – unless he's enormous and she's tiny, in which case the giant squid thing occasionally succeeds – is when you face the wall and he stands behind you. Place your palms on the flat surface to give yourself some leverage and arch your back so your bottom's sticking out towards him. He can then angle himself into you and hold onto your waist, or similarly, place his hands against the wall too. This way, he can use his penis or his hands to rub your clitoris and he can reach round to your breasts. Plus, most satisfyingly, nobody falls over. If you have a mirror alongside you, it works even better.

'Every man's favourite
position, the doggy…'

DOGGY STYLE

Every man's favourite position, the doggy offers total stimulation, a marvellous view of your bottom and fantasy-potential for both of you because you're not gazing directly into each other's eyes. You can either kneel on all fours with your back arched and your bottom pointing upwards invitingly, or leave your bottom thrust skywards while your head and shoulders lie comfortably on a pillow. Another variant is standing up and bracing your arms onto a bed or table. In all options, the basic key is that he's behind you and you're offering your bottom as a major beacon to sexual delight. It's a passionate, dirty position and every sex goddess keeps it in her repertoire for those times when you just don't feel like whispering sweet nothings (what do you mean, every time?).

THE CAT

From dog to cat… coming soon: 'the otter'. Just kidding. The cat position has nothing to do with fur or whiskers, unless you're willing to combine it with a role-play – and please, don't let me stop you. It is, in fact, the quick way of saying 'coital alignment technique', which sounds like a medical procedure, but is really a simple method of livening up your sex life. To do this, you lie on your back, and then he lies on top, puts his penis inside you, and inches upwards until his pelvis is level with your clitoris and he's very deeply inside you. At this point, he grinds in slow circles, placing delightful pressure on your clitoris. If you want to raise the excitement level more, clench and unclench your vagina with your internal pelvic-floor muscles (as if you wanted to stop a pee mid-flow) to bring him his own cat-like state of bliss.

'…bring him his own cat-like state of bliss.'

FACE TO FACE

Intimate and often impassioned, the face-to-face position is the best one for lovers who are deeply comfortable with one another. There are several variations – he sits on a chair, you straddle his lap; he kneels on the bed or floor and you kneel over him. If you're feeling particularly Tantric, he can sit cross-legged with you on his lap and you can cross your legs behind his back. You might be more tempted to pull faces or burst out laughing in this position, so you might feel more comfortable sticking with the less exotic poses. The benefits are that you can kiss, gaze into each other's eyes and establish a deep, emotional connection. Because the position is definitely about 'making love', there's nowhere to hide; the upside is that intimacy is intensified and the sex tends to be slower and meaningful. Not a good one to pick for a one-night stand, then…

SPOONS

This is the ideal sex position for lazy couples – and everyone's a lazy couple some time, say on a Sunday morning or just before dropping off to sleep on a Tuesday night. Being lazy doesn't mean you're not a sex goddess, just that you're not prepared to work all that hard to have a good time, and that's quite okay. 'Spoons' is so-named because your bodies fit together like spoons in a cutlery drawer, facing the same way. He lies behind you (obviously, if you lie behind him, it's never going to work) and you part your legs far enough to allow his penis entry. It helps if you bend forward a little, so that your bottom is shoved right up against him. Then he puts his arm around you, idly kisses your neck and plays with your breasts and you rock gently, to orgasm or to sleep – whichever happens first.

'...the dazzling clitoral stimulation of his pelvic bone against you.'

FACING AWAY

Occasionally known as the reverse cowgirl – you, the sex goddess, straddle him, but instead of facing his head you look at his feet. Not attractive, but hopefully the physical sensations make up for the view. You must be very careful not to bend his penis backwards, so when you lower yourself onto him, guide him in with your hand, then rock gently backwards and forwards – no thrusting up and down. You get the dazzling clitoral stimulation of his pelvic bone against you; he gets a superb view of your bottom and waist, and you can also reach under and stroke his balls. He can reach up and touch your breasts or grasp your waist, which is guaranteed to look tiny in this position.

HIS ORGASM

For a man, having an orgasm ought to be as simple as posting a letter in a slot – he shoots, he scores and he's done. But regardless of how much of a sex goddess you are, he may have problems. In fact, sometimes it's because you're such a sex goddess that he may not be able to cope with his own vast sexual desire for you, which can mean impotence, premature ejaculation or just sheer, god-awful performance anxiety. The commonest expression of male performance anxiety is being really, really bad at sex. So he'll mount you and thrust violently into you like a drone impregnating the Queen Bee, seconds before he dies. Or he'll give three little jabs of his penis and come before you've noticed he's in, or else he'll fail to get an erection and try to stuff it in anyway and hope you won't notice – you will, of course. There's only one way to deal with any and all of these symptoms and that's kindly and briskly. Gasping 'Oh my God, what's happened, is it me?' will help no one. Whereas a smile and a cuddle, perhaps with a brief comment such as, 'I'm tired too, let's do it later when we're not so exhausted,' will put the incident firmly in its place without destroying his fragile self-esteem.

*'Oh my God,
what's happened,
is it me?'*

*'He may not be able to
cope with his own vast
sexual desire for you.'*

Of course, if he thinks he's giving you a fantastic time, you can refer
to pages 52–53, which explain how to improve his sexual behaviour
while allowing him to think he did it all by himself. If the problem is a
recurring one, there are certain techniques that can be used.

BONING-UP TECHNIQUES

HERE ARE
THREE COMMON
PROBLEMS ON
THE ERECTION
FRONT AND WAYS
TO CIRCUMVENT
THEM.

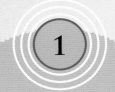

1

If premature ejaculation is nerves-based (if not, you should consult a doctor), you can train him out of this. You need the tried-and-tested stop-start technique, which means he enters you for one stroke, pulls out, waits for the excitement to subside, and then goes back in – like Jacques Cousteau after attaching a new oxygen tank. He stays in for a couple of strokes, exits before orgasm overtakes him, and repeats as necessary. You do need patience, but if he's stimulating you with his fingers in between, it shouldn't be too bad – quite enjoyable, in fact. You can also try the nurses' favoured technique: make a ring of your thumb and forefinger, and squeeze gently but firmly just underneath the head of his penis before he's about to come.

'…make a ring of your thumb and forefinger, and squeeze gently but firmly.'

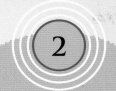

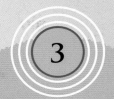

If he can't get an erection at all, try a slow, gentle blow job. And if that doesn't work, you can buy little devices called 'cock-rings', which fasten around the base of his penis and work to delay ejaculation, while maintaining an erection. However, if it's a regular problem, he needs a medical professional to cast an eye over the situation.

If he can get an erection, but can't orgasm, it's likely to be nerves. He should be able to relax in time as your relationship builds. Meanwhile, lay off the sex and see if he can come via a blow- or handjob. If so, it's probably only a matter of time before his sexual nerves wear off. If not, again he needs to consult a psychosexual therapist, which is not as scary as it sounds, to discover the emotional root of the problem.

MISMATCHED ORGASM SYNDROME

There's one problem that's enormously common – and as a sex goddess, it's almost certain that you'll be troubled by it at some point: mismatched orgasm syndrome (MOS). I made up the 'syndrome' bit, but it might as well be a medical fact.

You may have noticed, in your sexual adventures, that men tend to come first. In fact, unless you have a clitoris mounted on the outside of your body, which leads to enormously erotic feelings every time it's brushed against, you may have realized that they always come first – because you haven't got a penis and they have. The reasons why men orgasm more easily are far too complex to go into here, but basically if we don't come, we simply feel a bit fed up – whereas if they don't come, the human race grinds to a halt. So obviously, nature cares more about their orgasms.

Luckily, today's caring, sharing men like to make a woman come. We like coming. Yet to get his and her orgasms to coincide is like docking a space station blindfold. Unless you mutually masturbate, whereby you can slow down and he speeds up, having a simultaneous orgasm is unlikely. For most women, orgasming through intercourse means their clitoris must be consistently stimulated. For him to come, however, he needs to make jabbing, thrusting movements, which increase friction on the shaft of his penis – so it's all about the vagina. Which means, guess what?, that your paths to orgasm are totally different.

The easiest way to resolve this is for him to make you come first. Either with his hand, his tongue, by rubbing the tip of his penis against your clitoris or with a vibrator. Then, straight after, or even during, your orgasm, he can enter you and focus on his own excitement. Otherwise, he'll come first and fall asleep. It's a chemical thing – he can barely fight it. And you will be left, quite literally, high and dry. So it pays to concentrate on maximizing your orgasm.

MAKING THE MOST OF YOUR ORGASM

As you will know, if you've ever masturbated (yes, you have, I saw you), it's easy to come when you know what you're doing and nobody's watching you. It's much harder, however, when somebody else is second-guessing what you want and you're worrying about whether they're getting bored, or wondering if you're making funny noises and your stomach looks fat.

Inhibition is the enemy of orgasm, because to come you need to be fully relaxed, physically and mentally, and you aren't going to relax when your mind is playing a loop-tape entitled 'My Enormous Butt'.

'...practise a lot more to discover what fantasies and touches really work for you.'

If you're not used to orgasming alone, I suggest you practise a lot more – come on, it's no hardship – to discover what fantasies and touches really work for you. When you're with a new partner, don't put pressure on yourself to come quickly. It takes time for anyone to find out what turns you on, and while you can help and guide him, you may find your own nerves or uncertainty are preventing your orgasm. In this case, take the pressure off both of you by explaining to him that although you're having a great time, it just isn't going to happen tonight.

ALL-OVER STROKING

If you've been with your partner for a while, but you just can't shut up the internal voice that's bleating on about why it's taking so long and whether he really fancies you as much as his ex, you need to learn how to overcome your inner monologue, and all-over stroking is one of the best ways to do this.

> '*...sucking and licking your nipples while he touches you helps.*'

Light, feathery stroking is scientifically proven to access all the brain chemicals associated with nurturing, safety and comfort. When you're being stroked, it's hard not to relax. So a ten-minute period of caressing before he even gets near your clitoris will almost certainly speed up your eventual orgasm. It also helps if he's focused on you and doesn't look for a second as though he could be bored. So, sucking and licking your nipples while he touches you helps, as does kissing you rather than staring into space, appearing to fantasize about Scarlett Johansson and how much quicker than you she'd be. If he's getting the speed or pressure wrong, show him what you want, don't just lie there wincing silently. Never feel guilty about fantasizing – the vast majority of women can't come without it. Besides, what he doesn't know will never hurt him. Finally, it's not unusual to take up to an hour to reach orgasm, anything less and you're doing okay.

MULTIPLYING YOUR ORGASM

Does multiple orgasm exist? It depends on your definition of 'multiple'. Scientifically, it's generally assumed to mean 'more than one orgasm during a sexual encounter'. In which case, of course it does.

If your view of multiple orgasm, however, is based on porn movies, it means 'a wild, shuddering, over-acted orgasm that lasts for about three minutes and begins the moment a guy touches her'. In which case, get real, what do you think? It is possible, though, to have bigger, better orgasms without going into the ins and outs of Tantric sex, which promises orgasmic greatness. (We could, but we haven't got three years to study the ways of the Taoist masters, and you'd be so exhausted afterwards you would want a holiday, not a multiple orgasm.) The simplest techniques to multiorgasmic sex are 'the build-up' and 'the return'.

THE BUILD-UP

This does exactly what it says on the can. He strokes and rubs you closer and closer to the point of orgasm, and then breaks off, just as your breathing quickens and you think you can't bear it for him to stop. By the fourth or fifth time, you will be so worked up, you'll either crack him over the head with your heaviest vibrator out of sheer frustration or you'll tip over into the biggest orgasm you've ever had.

THE RETURN

This will guarantee greatness after you've had your first orgasm. Once you've calmed down, but the genital area is still sensitive, he should get down there and lick as gently and tenderly as he can. He must not touch your clitoris – it's too sensitive. But he can flick his tongue over the area all around it. After a while that orgasmic sensation will rebuild and when you do come, it will dwarf your previous orgasm like a tsunami crashing over a village pond. Honest.

FAKING IT

Sometimes the bitter truth is that even a sex goddess can't come. Whatever he does, however your vibrator wriggles and jiggles and tickles inside you, however many visions of Brad Pitt, oiled and ready for action, you conjure up, the internal workings are dead. You're tired, you're feeling angry, you can't switch your mind off tomorrow's work – whatever it is, it's just not happening. But the poor guy's trying so hard, wouldn't it be easier to keep him happy and pretend?

Well, not in my opinion. If faking makes you feel better, fine, keep practising your 'Oh… Oh! God! Yes!' noises, and hope they work. But in all truth, you're not so much being kind as dishonest. Because if you behave like you're having a great time when you're not, it can become a bit of a habit. Before you know it, there's a big faultline in your relationship: you're resentful, he's confused and all because you can't tell him how you're really feeling. It may be flattering to his ego to believe you're multiorgasmic at the flick of a switch, but it's a lot better for your relationship to be honest and admit that while it's not his fault (unless it is), you just aren't going to come right now.

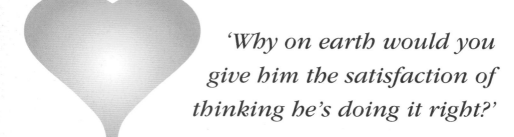

'Why on earth would you give him the satisfaction of thinking he's doing it right?'

If it's a one-night stand or a casual relationship, though, does it matter? Well, yes. Because really, why on earth would you give him the satisfaction of thinking he's doing it right when he so clearly isn't? You're a sex goddess, girl, not a groupie.

TOP FIVE WAYS TO ORGASM

There are many kinds of orgasms and many ways to have them. So feel free to think of more than five...

VIBRATOR

Possibly the easiest and quickest method of all. Switch it to the highest level, lie back and enjoy your filthiest fantasy. It'll all be over in five minutes, unless you want it to last, of course. You can use vibrators on your breasts and nipples, too. And while some women like to insert them, others prefer to rub the tip across their clitoris.

ORAL SEX

So long as he uses his tongue effectively and can touch your breasts at the same time, this should be a powerful and satisfying orgasm. If you can't come through oral sex, you may be nervous about what he's thinking. It's 99.9 per cent certain he's having a great time, so stop worrying.

MANUALLY

Correct use of his fingers on your clitoris, particularly when coupled with a finger sliding in and out of your vagina, should ensure an orgasm, but unless he knows your body well, it can take a while.

PENIS

If he grasps his penis and rubs the tip lightly over your clitoris, it should result in giddily orgasmic sensations for both of you. But he must not cheat and put it in. It also helps to use a bit of lube, to make it a smoother experience for both of you.

G-SPOT

If his fingers are long enough, he can insert one or two into your vagina and curl the tips over your pelvic bone on the front wall. Somewhere round here should be the G-spot, a spongy area the size of a small coin. If he can stroke it, it could result in a highly impressive orgasm.

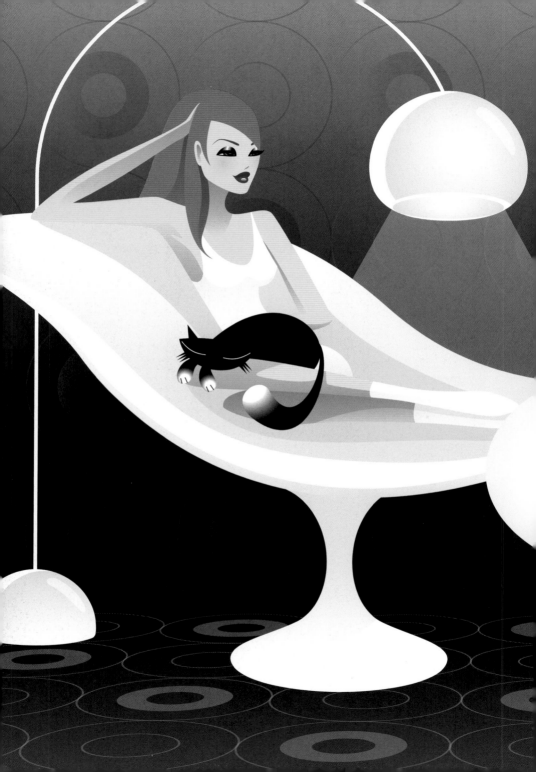

6 THE SINGLE GODDESS

'WHAT DO I WEAR IN BED? WHY, CHANEL NO. 5, OF COURSE.'

MARILYN MONROE

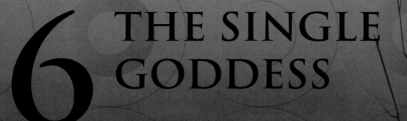

YOUR SEXY SELF

As we all know by now, feeling sexy comes down to self-esteem. But it's difficult to keep reminding yourself what a hot catch you are when you haven't seen yourself naked for six months and your pubic hair has been allowed to grow more Bornean rainforest than Brazilian beach. So the first thing to do is to take a good look in the mirror. I know, I understand, the very idea of seeing The Stomach under harsh, unforgiving bathroom lights, or twisting round to view The Butt in its full, baggy glory, may not be quite the instant turn-on you're hoping for. In which case, you need to sit down first and make a list – mental or otherwise – of all the nice things your lovers have ever said about your body. If they never have (what were you doing with them in the first place?), then list the parts of your body you're most proud of yourself.

'Feeling sexy comes down to self-esteem.'

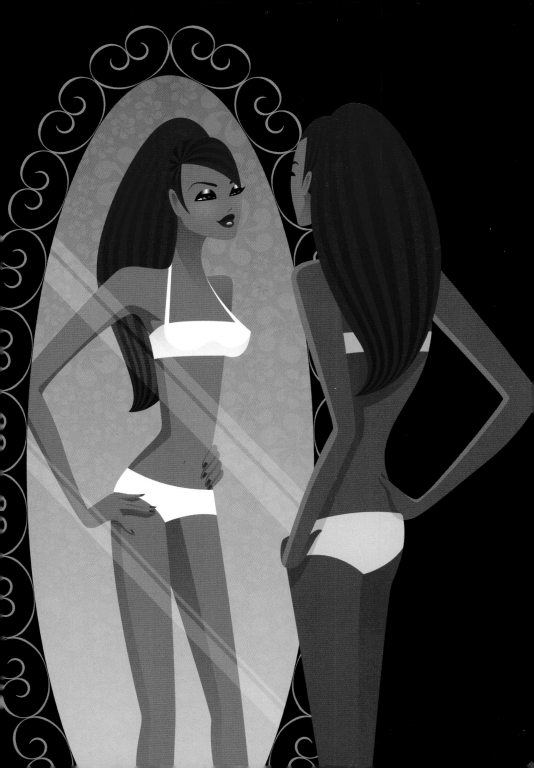

MIRROR, MIRROR

With the list in mind, turn the lights right down, as low as you like (if you're really insecure, a low-wattage bulb glowing feebly from another room is perfectly acceptable), and strip down to your best underwear or full nudity, whichever you prefer, in front of a full-length mirror. Make sure you've got make-up on and your hair's brushed – we're aiming to see what a new lover would view, not a vision of what humankind might look like after a meteor hits Earth – and remember your mother's advice about posture. Shoulders back, stomach in. You will also find that rather than standing square on, if you balance your weight slightly on one hip and turn three-quarters to the mirror, you'll look instantly thinner. For a masterclass in this, see Elizabeth Hurley in any photograph taken throughout her entire career.

Now, obviously, there's going to be stuff here you don't like, however you stand. You're a woman and it's in your job description not to like everything about the way you look. However, your challenge is to focus on at least six things about your face and body that you're fond of, and ignore the rest. When men look at sex goddesses, they don't think, 'Hmm, great bust, but really, her ankles are a little chunky.' They simply home in instantly on the bits that are best presented – and besides, even if your ankles look like redwood trunks, that's what boots are for.

'…balance your weight slightly on one hip and turn three-quarters to the mirror, you'll look instantly thinner.'

TOUCHING YOURSELF

The whole purpose of this exercise is to see yourself as an appreciative man would see you, not as a critical diet doctor. And once you've located the good parts, you need to wake them up by the power of touch. You can do this in front of the mirror or lie down for a more comfortable exploration. It's a simple matter of caressing yourself in a way that feels sensual. So, if you do hate your tummy, ignore it. Focus on your lovely ankles or your swan-like neck and stroke yourself there instead.

> *'It's a simple matter of caressing yourself in a way that feels sensual.'*

Admittedly, you may feel a bit of a fool writhing around, fondling your own kneecaps, but you need to learn to accept yourself as a sensual being. If you don't do this, then every time you leave your home, you will be projecting the words, 'Don't fancy me, I'm repulsive' in giant letters above your head. Strangely enough, men will pick up on that, and steer well clear. Training yourself to accept and enjoy your own body will change your projected sentiment to 'Whoooh, check this out, baby', or words to that effect. So there is method in the madness, believe me.

Once you've had a good feel of all your most impressive bits – and there's no hurry, you can play with your breasts for as long as you like, men would if they had them – it's time to move on to what certain coy people like to call 'self-pleasure'. Mastery of masturbation can do wonders for your sex-goddess status. It makes you feel great, it gives you that glowing, sexy look that you usually only get from fantastic first-night sex and it boosts your confidence faster than a Viagra-Prozac cocktail. And all from a flick of the wrist.

MASTURBATION

Obviously, it doesn't make you go blind. In fact, masturbation has all sorts of benefits, such as boosting your immune system (and better than nettle tea, too), enhancing your sense of wellbeing and making you more likely to win the lottery. Okay, I made that last one up, but it's still pretty good. Most women masturbate, but don't talk about it. Just because the subject is as carefully concealed as our clitoris, doesn't mean it's shameful.

So throw out all those bad-girl feelings of dirtiness, shame, embarrassment and wickedness. Or pay a good therapist to help you with this. If your mother told you God would strike you down for your exploratory childhood fiddling, I have one question, 'Are you still here?' And if anyone told you that 'self-abuse' was evil, ask yourself, 'Has an orgasm ever started a war?' Okay, Helen of Troy, but that wasn't masturbation, so it doesn't count. Forget your guilt and welcome woman's best friend: your clitoris. Get to know it, because it's time you had some fun.

Occasionally, women insist that they 'don't know' if they've had an orgasm; if you have, you'll know. Because, while your clitoris will stand any amount of frenzied rubbing before you come, afterwards it just wants to curl up in a ball and be left alone, and that's not to mention the waves of excitement and release of tension. So actually, you probably do know. The more you masturbate, the more you'll come to understand what works for you and the sexier you'll feel. And when you do have a partner, you'll be in a better position to explain what you want in bed.

'Forget your guilt and welcome woman's best friend: your clitoris.'

HOW TO SELF-AMUSE

Self-amusing is a much more accurate description than self-abusing, particularly for a sex goddess. So to keep your sex drive well oiled, even in fallow times, masturbate whenever you feel the urge. Well, not when you're on the bus, I mean in private. Though there's no harm in sneaking to the bathroom at work for a quickie, so long as you can do it silently. If you're not sure how, it's really very simple.

1. Find somewhere private – if you have housemates, put the chain on the door and if you have parents or, even worse, children who may burst in, buy a deadlock bolt for your bedroom door. That's how much you don't want to be caught masturbating, and not because it's wrong, just because it's private.

2. Now take your knickers (panties) off – you'll never get anywhere with a bunch of fabric cutting off your route to victory. Find a hand mirror and make sure the room is well-lit.

3. Use your fingers to part your labia and have a good look. If you've never become familiar with this part of your anatomy, the little lentil-shaped thing at the top is your clitoris, the tiny hole in the middle is your urethra and the big hole at the base is your vagina. If you're not turned on, just stroke gently around your vagina until it gets slightly wet, and then use your lubricated fingertip to circle your clitoris. And if you still find the skin dragging, lubricating jelly will ease things.

4. Try out different pressures and movements until you feel strange and undeniable stirrings of excitement, then just keep going. Some women like to touch their nipples (well, one nipple) at the same time, while others enjoy pushing a vibrator or another finger in and out of their vaginas. Some like to lie on a pillow and gyrate their hips against it; other women will only use a vibrator on their clitoris. Basically, the end result – orgasm – is the same. You may find you come a great deal faster via masturbation than you do with a man.

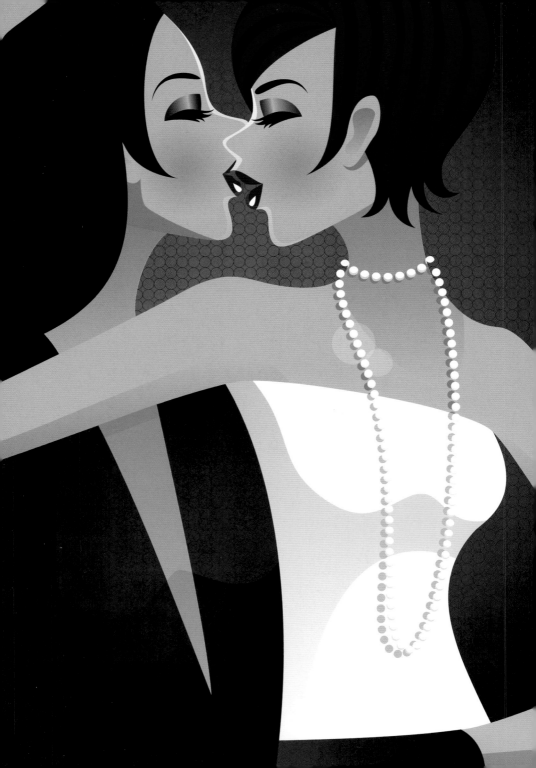

BEING BI-CURIOUS

In recent years, increasing numbers of apparently straight women have been expressing their bisexual curiosity. We can assume it was always there, though it's more acceptable to explore your Sapphic side today – what with female celebrities kissing each other every time they need column inches, gay and lesbian singers crossing to the mainstream, magazines such as *Diva* 'for the lesbian in you', and every other film, TV soap and drama series featuring a lesbian or bisexual character.

There are even websites devoted to bi-curious girls, which allow you to chat with other women like you. All of which is a complex way of saying that if you fancy other women, or simply fantasize about sex with them, that doesn't mean you're a lesbian and you have to undergo a major lifestyle change and come out to your parents and your boss, waving rainbow flags. It just means you're comfortable with your sexuality, and there's a hell of a lot of pretty women out there.

If you'd like to turn your curiosity into action, you can go about this in two ways – get drunk with an open-minded female friend, and see how she reacts when you kiss her – or the easy way. The first is certainly an option, but as with threesomes, orgies and similar, recruiting close friends into sexual exploration is an emotional minefield. What if she hates it? What if you're too embarrassed to cope afterwards? What if she loves it and falls for you, when you were just interested in checking out how her breasts felt? So, the second option may be safer, which is to locate a women-only or 'lesbian and bi-curious' club night in your local area, and get along there for a chat and a dance. If that's way too scary for you, locate a lesbian-run social group for the confused and bi-curious, on the Internet or in person, and make your approach. It might turn out you're not as keen as you thought you were when faced with the reality, or it may be the beginning of a whole new lifestyle. Just don't tell men or you'll be doomed to a lifetime of 'Can I watch?' requests.

THE SENSUAL WORLD

Just feeling sexy isn't enough for a true sex goddess. Your whole world should be appealingly sensual. Floating about in silks and satins and masturbating more often than a 15-year-old boy on a Playboy shoot will not work if your living environment is a mound of discarded takeout cartons, old newspapers and dirty underwear. To live as a sex goddess, your surroundings must be sexed-up too. If your living space looks more like a dentist's waiting room (harsh overhead lights, furniture pushed against walls) than a Turkish opium den, it needs fixing. When you open your door, you want to feel that your place expresses who you are, whether that's sporty and sexy, or girly and sexy, or any other permutation of sexy you care to name.

'To live as a sex goddess, your surroundings must be sexed-up too.'

Colours that enhance the sensuality of a room include reds, pinks, oranges, browns and golds. Try black, but use it sparingly with pink or red. White is relaxing and an all-white room can offer a feeling of deep calm and peace, which can be highly sensual – but if you overdo it, it can look like an operating room. Liven up your walls with colourful framed pictures or prints – original art is more personal and dynamic than the same photo-print two million others bought. It doesn't have to cost anything – most of us are capable of making something attractive to hang on the wall, even if it's just a selection of leaves in a frame. You can even hang your loveliest dress, scarf or jewellery on the wall, to admire and inspire.

'Candles make everyone look at least six times more attractive.'

Also vital is lighting; harsh, overhead light is the bitter enemy of sensuality. Unless you're involved in painstaking surgical work or are searching for a lost earring, you don't actually need the relentless blaze of white overhead light. At least three lamps, placed strategically around the room, will create a comforting and attractive glow. Candles, too, make everyone look at least six times more attractive (I'm sure this is scientific fact) and twice as thin. Lava lamps, with their slow-moving, retro vibe, are ideal sensual lighting; spotlights, which reveal every flaw no matter how well disguised, are not.

As for texture, if your furniture is looking less than perfect, invest in some throws made from fake fur or velvet. Obviously, you don't want the place to look like a bear trapper's cabin, so don't go overboard on the nylon wolf-fur, but do think about texture as much as visual appeal. The bed will benefit from a pile of pillows and a velvet or satin bedspread, but if you have a penchant for dainty floral prints, do try and wean yourself off them. Sex goddesses don't live in a herbaceous border, on the whole.

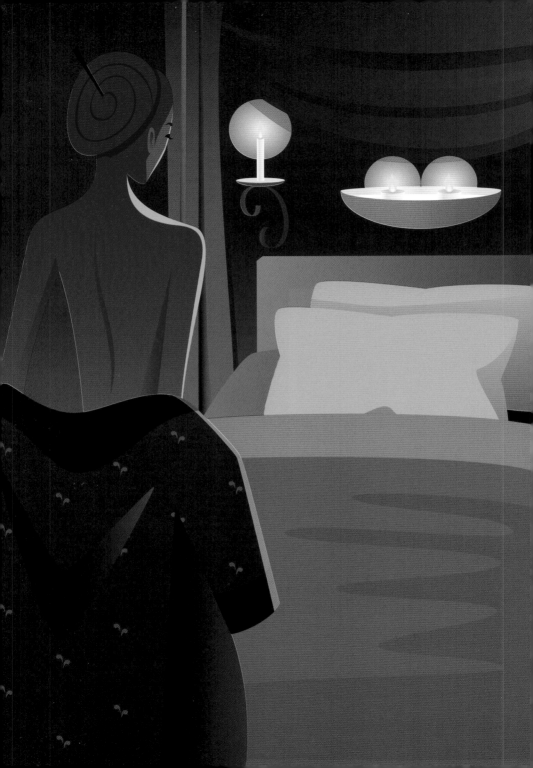

'Try sensual scented candles or liberal sprays of expensive perfume.'

If you smoke or have animals, you'll need the air to smell a little nicer. Personally, I think air fresheners smell like the devil's pantyliners. Far more sensual are scented candles, real flowers and the old favourite sell-your-house smells of real coffee and baking bread (put a market-bought loaf in the oven – who'll know?). If, like me, you're a bit of a slut, you may simply choose to disguise the dirty washing with liberal sprays of expensive perfume, which also have the bonus of making your house smell like an eighteenth-century French whore's boudoir. And all you need then is a reasonable level of tidiness. We're not talking anal neatness, just the sense that if you put something down, it won't immediately be obscured by dustballs and a top layer of mould. Basically, living like a sex goddess is all about making your environment as desirable as you are. Which is, of course, very.

'Living like a sex goddess is all about making your environment as desirable as you are.'

TOP TEN WAYS TO SEX UP YOUR SINGLE LIFE

VIBRATOR

Every girl's 'other' best friend. You need a vibrator to provide quick, easy orgasms at the flick of a switch. Try the small 18cm (7in) three-speed type. It's subtle, relatively stylish and does the job.

PERFUME

Always smell nice, it doesn't matter if you're not going anywhere. A spray of scent on your pulse points will clothe you in a sensual waft of delightful fragrance all day long. Try lots of brands before you decide which is 'your' signature scent.

UNDERWEAR

Even if the only time anyone's going to see your underwear is if you're taken to the hospital after an accident, you should still make sure it's nice. It doesn't have to match exactly, but black knickers and bras should go together. Wear silky, lacy, sensual underwear and you will feel good about yourself, whatever you wear on top.

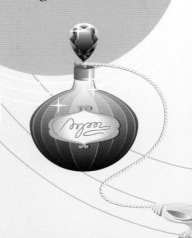

MUSIC

The deafening silence of singledom is not pleasant, so get into the habit of putting on music when you're alone. It can enhance your mood faster than any drug. Download some feel-good tunes, and whatever your mood, you'll have suitable sounds for 'Yeah! I'm Single,' 'No One Loves Me,' and 'But I'm Sexy Anyway'.

CHAMPAGNE

I'm not advocating drinking alone (well, I occasionally might), but it's always helpful to have a bottle of champagne in the fridge. Like the emergency alarm on trains, it's simply nice to know it's there. You can open it after a terrible day, great news or just on a wet weekend – and what's more, you can then think of yourself as the type of woman who always has champagne in the refrigerator.

SILK SHEETS

Cotton sheets are all very well, but for true sensuality, you need one set of silk sheets. If there's no one to cuddle up to, wrapping your body in warm silk is the next-best thing – and when there is, it's unlikely he'll complain either. However, don't take this to mean that anything warm and comforting is acceptable in bed. Grown women with a herd of fluffy toys on the pillow don't look like sex goddesses, they look scary.

CAT

While you're self-assured and independent, sometimes it's nice to have someone to talk to. To stop you jabbering away to yourself like a lunatic, consider the perfect sex goddess companion: a cat. Dogs are too much like men – messy, eager and constantly in need of attention – whereas a cat simply slinks about, dispensing affection and warmth when it feels like it and wandering off to sleep when it doesn't. Plus they look good, and if you can get one that matches your hair or your interior décor, so much the chicer.

HAIR

Just because you haven't got anyone to run fingers through your hair right now, doesn't mean you should neglect it. To maintain your sex-goddess stance, while single or coupled up, a great haircut is essential. Pay as much as you can afford and ask for a style that can be maintained easily. Well-groomed hair that looks healthy and touchable will make you feel gorgeous.

SHOES

All sex goddesses are elevated
to heavenly status by shoes. Their
patron saint may be Victoria Beckham
with her Louboutins, but any girl can goddess
herself up with a pair of killer stilettos, even if
they come from a thrift shop and cost a whole lot
less than $600. They lengthen your legs, push out
your bottom and make you walk like Marilyn – who,
rumour has it, used to shave a little off one heel to
give herself that sexy sway. If you really want to go
for it, invest in a pair of porn shoes – towering
heels, ankle straps and only worn by naked
women who are about to bend over; these
shoes are the ultimate in slut-wear, but
in a good way.

NEGLIGEE

No one looks good in a
towelling dressing gown (bathrobe).
It's warm, it's cosy, but it ain't sexy. What
you need is the kind of loungewear you
see in Hollywood movies – the sheer, almost
see-through negligee (see also pages 68–71).
It wisps around your body, drapes over your
curves and enhances your every movement.
Get one in silk or satin, which warms
to the temperature of your body, and
slink around the house – the only
problem will be bothering to
get dressed at all.

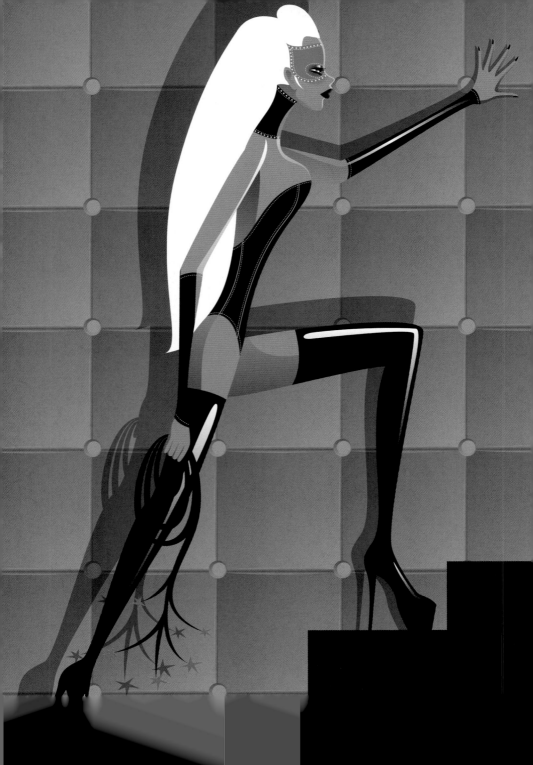

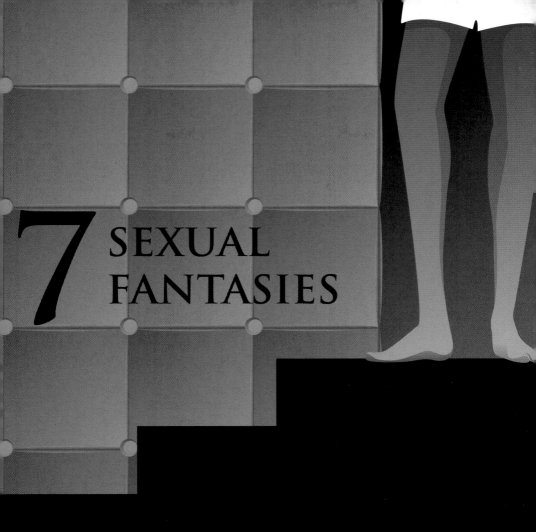

7 SEXUAL FANTASIES

'EVER NOTICE THAT "WHAT THE HELL" IS ALWAYS THE RIGHT DECISION?'

At the beginning of a relationship, sex is great, and that's without any props, aids or spicing-up. But after a while, the old naked one-two starts to feel a little dull. At that point, any sex goddess will do one of two things. She'll either leave him and go on to enjoy three energetic months with somebody new, or she'll introduce 'Fantasy Sex' into the relationship to ensure that their lovemaking stays fresh, funky and positively unforgettable for many more months, possibly even years, to come. Everybody has sexual fantasies and while some are for entirely private consumption only – the ones involving other men who are sexier than him, for example – there are plenty worth sharing.

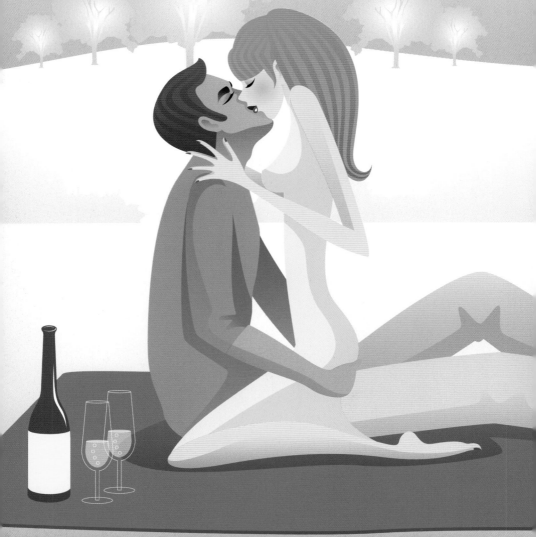

SHARING FANTASIES

First rule: if you can't take the truth, don't ask the question. So if you're keen to ask, 'Do you ever think about other women when we're having sex?', realize that there's at least a 50 per cent chance the answer's going to be 'yes'. And if he asks you (about men or women), weigh up your answer carefully to avoid weeks of gloomy silences and hurt glances. While couples often claim that they can tell each other anything, they're only smug because they don't know the half of it. Good fantasies to share are basic erotic ideas, or those that involve the two of you. Bad ones to mention are fantasies concerning others, such as ex-partners, family members and best friends. It's not that there's anything wrong with a healthy fantasy life involving your boss and your partner's brother, it's just that your partner probably doesn't want to know.

That said, you can adapt almost any fantasy and make it palatable to share with your partner – it's a simple matter of taking it slowly, revealing a detail at a time and leaving out the questionable dream lover. Talking about your fantasies together means you get an insight into what turns each other on (and why). It also considerably boosts the chances that you'll actually get to enact them, if the same ideas turn you both on. Beginning the conversation, however, isn't always simple. Blurting out, 'So, what are you thinking about?' at the point of orgasm won't allow him to open up gradually and sensitively. He's more likely to shout 'Tits!' and then regret it later. If you want to uncover his deepest desires, and reveal yours, the best way to instigate the discussion is while you're in bed, but still coherent. Perhaps a little stroking may take place to get you both in the mood, but anything more passionate makes it hard to talk.

Broach the topic with a question such as, 'Do you ever think about doing it outside?' If he pulls away from you, horrified, and stammers, 'But the police would shout at us,' then perhaps don't take this any further. Any sort of encouraging response can lead to, 'Where would you like to do it with me?' and 'What exactly would we do?' Before you know it, you're telling him exactly how you've always fancied having sex on the battlements of a windswept castle, dressed as Anne Boleyn – or whatever. When he tells you his own fantasies, don't exclaim, 'But that's so basic and dull.' Most men don't enjoy the same wild, flowery imaginations as most women. For them, a simple 'she's wearing stockings' will generally suffice as a trigger, while women often like to create a cast of thousands entirely in period dress with a full script and a lighting technician before they can even begin to get turned on.

DRESSING UP AND ROLE-PLAY

Once you've established the ideas that work for both of you, as a sex goddess and sex god, you may like to put them into practice. Not really hiking up to the battlements, silly; we're talking about role-play, the art of pretending. It used to be called 'playing', but we're all adults now.

Role-play is a fantastic way to add a new dimension to your sex life, which can offer all the benefits of infidelity without any of the guilt or pain. All you need to do is decide on your fantasy roles (you can swap around any time). Collect together an adult dressing-up box, containing such items as hats, scarves, a feather boa, spectacles or even a nurse's outfit. Let your imagination run free, but remember, often you only need one item to suggest a role – you don't need the full TV drama props department.

A basic script helps, but don't make it too involved or get in-depth about subplots and motivation. A few dialogue lines to get you in the mood will do. Try 'Oh no, my car's broken down' (though not if you're being Anne Boleyn), 'I feel so warm, I can't think why', 'Where exactly does it hurt, Sir?' and so on. Good role-plays with strong dramatic parts for both of you include teacher and pupil, nurse or doctor and patient, businessman or -woman and interviewee, lady/master of the manor and servant, and damsel in distress and helpful stranger. If you're filming it, use a tripod and try not to laugh; also remember not to spend too long chatting and adjusting your costume. The whole point is to have sex, and role-play often helps couples to shed their inhibitions faster than a bottle of vodka, because you're only acting, so you can say and do whatever you want.

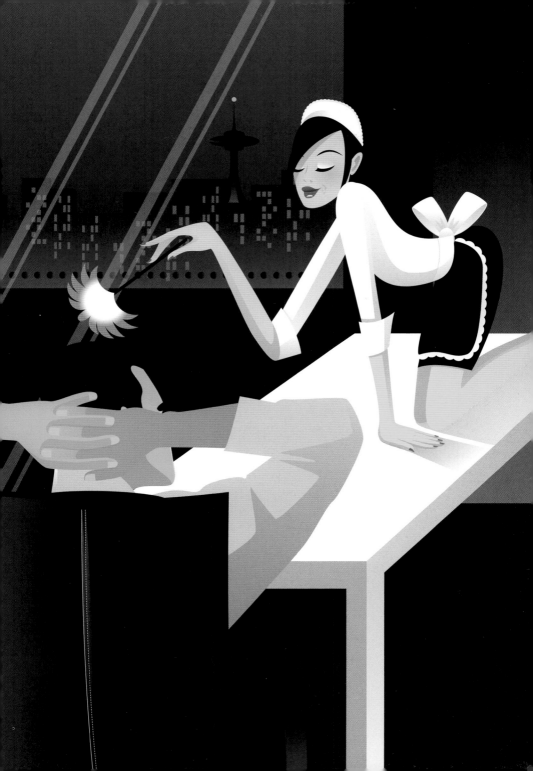

MASTURBATION

How far you go sexually is, of course, entirely up to you. But the genuine goddess has a fairly full repertoire, purely because it makes life interesting. And if you never try it, how do you know whether you like it or not?

One area of experimentation, which never used to be mentioned, but is now regularly discussed, is anal sex. Men generally love it because it's a very tight fit and it's thoroughly dirty (in the sexual sense that is). Often women aren't so keen because, for them, it's mainly painful and they worry that it's going to be dirty in an entirely different sense. Some women find the whole idea unnerving, and it's certainly a type of sex that depends on trust. They may feel degraded or distressed by the sheer physical intimacy of it, and if so, it's important to talk first. If you're doing it as a gesture of love, make sure he knows that, or he may expect a night of filthy passion and you'll be weeping into the pillow.

Ironically, men have a prostate gland up their anus, which produces pleasingly erotic sensations when stimulated. Women, sadly, do not. So the pleasure of anal sex is largely mental excitement generated by doing something 'dirty', although some women do enjoy the sensation of fullness, particularly if they also have something (a finger, a vibrator) in their vagina at the same time.

'...if you never try it, how do you know whether you like it or not?'

'You should be very turned on first – it won't work from a standing start.'

If you decide to give anal a whirl, there are certain basic rules for making the experience as pleasant as possible. First, it helps if he hasn't got a massive penis – though don't point this out to him. Whatever size it is, you need a lot of lubrication around your anus and all over his penis, which will be wearing a condom. Anal skin tears very easily, so hello pain and infections if you aren't careful. You can get heavy-duty condoms for anal sex, though you might prefer to order them via the Internet.

You should be very turned on first – it won't work from a standing start. Unless all your muscles are thoroughly relaxed, it'll just feel like someone trying to wedge a grapefruit into a keyhole. Once you're in the mood, the best position is doggy style. That way, he can see exactly what he's doing. He needs to enter you very, very slowly, 1cm (½in) at a time. Make it clear before he begins to thrust that violent plunging is out; only gentle, slow thrusts are acceptable.

When he pulls out, he must not touch your vagina with his penis because bacteria can be transferred. Apart from that, you're fine. Anything you heard about anal prolapse isn't true – you'd have to do it with an entire rugby team for three days' straight to cause that kind of problem, and we all know you're not that kind of girl.

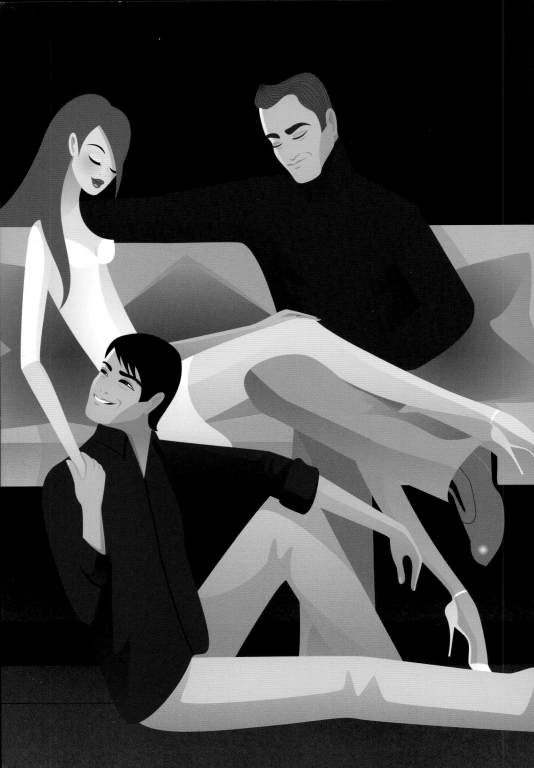

THREESOMES
AND ORGIES

This is where even the sexiest goddess glances behind her in nervous, Scooby Doo fashion, as she prepares to step further into the deserted ghost train that is threesomes and orgies. While they are the mainstay of porn and a hugely popular fantasy, the reality can be scarier than a whole bunch of skeletons. It's not that they aren't enjoyable – physically they can be great, which is why there are so many clubs and parties offering a modern take on the old 1970s sport of swinging – this time without the car keys and the droopy 'taches. But emotionally – well, hold on tight.

Recruiting someone else to have sex with you and your partner is like sticking your hand in a crocodile pen for the buzz. It might be exciting, but it can all end in disaster. If it's a female friend, there's the jealousy issue – is she better in bed than me? Has he always fancied her? Will he want her more than me? What if they start doing it behind my back? If it's a male friend, ditto for him. And if it's a stranger culled from the Internet or a local swinger's night, you know nothing about them or their strange sexual diseases, or even, possibly, their loving partner and three kids back home.

Then there's the possibility that you'll like it too much and suddenly, two-person sex won't seem anything like as much fun. Or you'll fall in love with them or they'll fall in love with you, and you can never see them again without blowing your relationship sky-high. Of course, there is a slim possibility that you'll all have a great time sexually, remain healthy, mutually supportive adults throughout, and agree to do it every so often on special occasions, while happily returning to normality in between. And there's a possibility that the crocodile won't feel very hungry. But it's not very likely.

If you do go ahead, despite everything, always observe threesome etiquette, which states that no person must feel left out. Two people getting it on while another watches miserably from the sidelines is not a threesome, it's a floorshow. Wondering how to get started? Well, I'm tempted to say that if you can't get that far on your own, you probably shouldn't be attempting it at all. But if you're really stuck, try strip poker with forfeits.

Oddly enough, orgies are actually a safer bet emotionally, if you can cope with the sight of your partner amid a writhing pit of nubile lovelies. Having said that, most swingers aren't that lovely, so if you are going to try it, you may want to investigate the possibility of joining a very exclusive, members-only club that only permits beautiful people to swing. Otherwise you may be stuck with 'Over-40s Night' at Xanadu Blue, above the Chinese takeaway.

Of course, if you are going to swing, never, ever, swing in any direction without a condom and never do anything you feel unsure about, just because your partner swears it's his (or her) greatest fantasy. Let them keep it as a fantasy and then you retain your self-respect and mental wholeness. You're a sex goddess, remember, not a sex toy.

SADOMASOCHISM AND BONDAGE

S&M is about giving and receiving pain, domination and submission. But the roster of experiences that fall beneath that heading range from a mild tap on the bottom to being hung from a hook and ritually flogged by a gimp-masked master. Most of us don't want to go as far as that but that doesn't mean we don't want to experiment, trying on the sub (submissive) and dom (dominant) personas for size.

Sadists get turned on by inflicting pain, while masochists enjoy receiving it. But that doesn't mean you can't swap if you're not sure which one works for you. For some, there's a thin line between pain and pleasure. The nerves are stimulated by both and if your brain makes a connection between pain and excitement, this can quickly translate into desire. There are basic elements to S&M, so if you're interested, read on – you may as well do it right, rather than attempting a flogging with a bent coat hanger and wondering why it's not much fun.

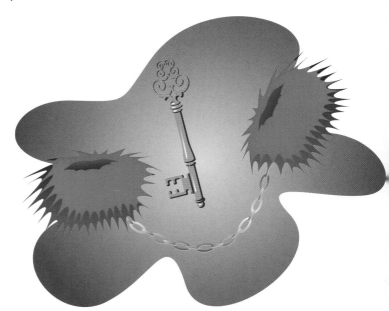

LEATHER, RUBBER AND OTHER CLOTHING

S&M clothes are all about power, so black is usually the colour of choice. Skintight PVC and leather are also popular, as is specially constructed underwear hung with chains and studs. The erotic ideas of restraint and bondage are usually apparent, too, and shiny high heels are obligatory, the more kitten-skewering the better. Blindfolds are also useful, but you can improvise out of silk scarves. Fetish shops stock entire ranges, from lacy basques to studded and buckled helmets, so your particular sartorial fancy shouldn't be hard to find. Some S&M-ers swear by leather, because it has the feel of warm skin and the smell can be erotic. Others prefer the modern stretch of PVC, while still more insist that rubber is the only true S&M clothing. Whether you want jackboots and a studded pouch, or a high heels-and-stockings combo, you can adapt your favourite parts of the S&M look and discard the rest. Fetish-wear generally makes women – particularly sex goddesses – look tall, thin and menacingly powerful, which can only be a good thing.

PROPS AND ACCESSORIES

The committed S&M-er may have an enormous box of tricks dedicated purely to hanging, strapping, thrashing and slapping. However, for the weekend hobbyist – or the sex goddess who just wants to spice up her life – there are only a few basics required. The chief accessory is a set of handcuffs, and the fluffy versions are much more comfortable. The main points to remember are: don't lose the key, whatever you do, and don't leave anyone handcuffed to anything for long, or they'll faint from restricted blood flow.

'The chief accessory is a set of handcuffs, and the fluffy versions are much more comfortable.'

The most comfortable 'cuffed' position is with the hands in front of the body, but if that's not bondage-porn enough for you both, you can cuff your partner to a piece of furniture (like the bed). If you're lying down, avoid cuffing behind the back; hands stuck underneath the bottom is unpleasant, rather than arousing. If handcuffs seem a little hardcore, use bondage tape (often available from sex shops in black or pink), which unpeels easily but does the job.

You can gag each other if you want, but never put anything tight around someone's neck. You may also wish to invest in a small whipping device. A leather cat o'nine tails is good, as it provides the requisite swishing noise, feels suitably naughty when whacked against bare buttocks and looks the part. You can buy a full whip, but they're difficult to wield accurately and the danger is that you might do infinitely more damage than you ever intended to. There's always the riding crop option (and they provide a fair slap), but again this can be agonizing if wielded harshly. Order a few types from the Internet and send back the scariest – or keep them, depending on your point of view.

'Order a few types from the Internet and send back the scariest.'

Nipple clamps and similar accessories are also an option. Today you can have any part of your body pierced, clamped or electrified, and S&M-ers frequently do. If you are considering this, make sure you go to a reputable piercing establishment. Do your research thoroughly first, too – if you don't like it, it's a bit late once you've had a metal post shot through your clitoris.

LESSONS IN SAFETY

Of course when you're incorporating pain, bondage and helplessness into your sex games, there's always a danger that something can go wrong. If you're mid-role-play and shout, 'No, stop!', there's every chance your partner will simply assume you're throwing yourself into character, and carry on. That's why S&M fans have a 'safe word', which can only be used in the context of 'end the game now' or 'stop what you're doing'. The word is usually something incongruous like 'teapot'.

Both S&M and bondage require a high level of trust, and anyone who's ever been sexually or emotionally abused should be particularly careful. What's a fun power game to one person can easily be a damaging reminder of a painful past experience to another. Make sure you are happy with what's going on at all times, don't allow anyone you don't know and trust to tie you up, and if you feel uncomfortable, say so. You should only ever play these games with someone you trust. One-night stands are not the time to put yourself in a position of vulnerability. And if your new lover seems a bit too keen to slap you in handcuffs, you may want to wonder why.

EXHIBITIONISM AND VOYEURISM

Exhibitionists like to reveal themselves, or get caught having sex. For them, the thrill comes from being viewed. So if you're a sex goddess who happens to be an exhibitionist, you need to make sure you don't get arrested – or worse, assaulted. Walking around semi-naked is out, as is having sex in front of the window, which could cause offence to passers-by. Find a way to demonstrate your desires safely.

Outdoor sex can be relatively safe, but it's illegal in many countries and can count as public obscenity. Well, you may think you're a thing of beauty and a joy forever, but the policeman might disagree. So if you do crave risky exhibitionist sex, choose a deserted beach or a secluded wood over a nightclub dance-floor, and an empty alleyway over a main road.

That way, you still get the buzz of knowing someone might see you, but it's less likely, at least. It is also essential to know the legal restrictions of the country you are in, as your perfect romantic break might end up in prison. The other, more failsafe, way to indulge your exhibitionism is to film yourselves making love – or just alone, stripping or masturbating. That way, your lovemaking won't be seen by anyone but you, though you will still get the excitement of seeing yourself on screen and you can even pretend you're turning on the entire nation. If you really want to, you can send your film to one of the porn companies specializing in 'real couples' – and just hope your parents aren't racier than you thought when it comes to spicing up their own love life via mail-order video. If you go down this route, consider drawing up a contract which ensures that your partner can't post you on the Internet in all your glory or distribute your image to his 500 closest friends. If you're in any doubt, you can consult a solicitor (attorney) and take advice on making it legal and binding.

> *'...the Internet is just bursting with web-cam couples dying to be watched.'*

For voyeurs life is more difficult (isn't it always?), because watching other people without their knowledge is, naturally enough, a criminal offence. However, there are private clubs that allow voyeurs to meet exhibitionists – now there's a match made in heaven – and watch them writhe around. But if that's too scary, the Internet is just bursting with web-cam couples dying to be watched, though make sure it's a secure site and they're not going to get your financial details and wipe your account. Be careful, too, not to follow any questionable links involving 'young and sexy' girls, or the police might make a questionable link to you.

SEX TOYS

Strictly speaking, sex toys aren't all that experimental, given that nowadays a good 50 per cent of women own one. But they're definitely worth including in your sex-goddess repertoire – and not just for times when your boyfriend's out of town. One vibrator is fine, but there's so many shapes and sizes available, it's more fun to have a few. A good selection would be a normal 18cm (7in) three-speed. This is good for holding against your clitoris when he's inside you, and can also buzz pleasantly against the shaft of his penis. Then you need a waterproof toy for shower- and bath-based sex – a good model is 'I Rub My Duckie', which is – as you'd suspect – a vibrator cunningly disguised as a rubber duck. You could also use the cock-ring/vibrating attachment sort, which is a soft rubber ring that fits round the base of his penis with a projecting section of nodules that lie against your clitoris, providing a constant buzz as he grinds away – so convenient. You could also choose a lipstick-shaped one that you can discreetly carry in your bag – or the old classic 'Rabbit' vibrator with all the jiggling balls, for those times when your orgasm is all that matters.

Then there are the more esoteric toys – the anal beads, for example, which you place up his bottom (use lubrication at this point, and don't argue) and whip out at the moment of orgasm to stimulate his prostate. Or the 'Tongue Joy', which slips over the tongue to sex up oral with an extra buzz. The best way to choose the ingredients of your personal sex-goddess toy box is to take a tour of the sex shop websites or in person in the increasingly female-friendly new sex shops (see resources on page 160).

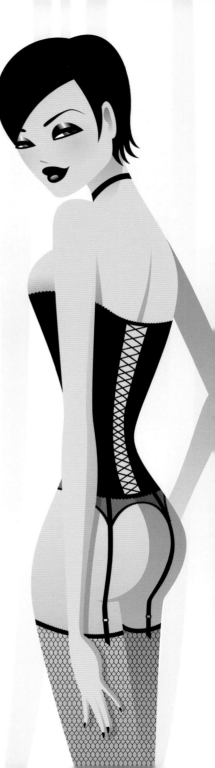

TOP TEN
GODDESS PROPS

1. LEATHER GLOVES

Texturally exciting for stroking and handjobs,
leather gloves also add a dangerous frisson to
S&M sexual encounters.

2. HANDCUFFS

Try the fluffy ones, or silk-lined if you prefer,
and make sure you can lock and unlock them
easily. The metal policeman's kind can bite
unpleasantly, but you might find that exciting.

3. VIBRATOR

Every sex goddess should have one. Work
out what you want it for – clitoris, vagina,
penis-substitute, double penetration with his
penis or simply a gentle buzzing sensation –
and supplement your box of delights with as
many types as you like.

4. LUBE

A bedroom (or elsewhere) essential, a tube of
lubrication is needed when foreplay just isn't
doing the trick, you're tired and stressed and
you're experimenting with some anal sex (see
pages 128–129). Just a drop will be enough to
replicate your natural secretions and it's more
pleasant if you warm it in your palms first.
You can also use it to ease your handjobs –
it'll speed them up remarkably.

5. VIDEO CAMERA

Cheaper technology means that anyone can make their own private porn film. Get a tripod, press 'record' and away you go. And if you want to make a Victorian porn film, simply turn the dial to 'sepia' for a strangely erotic time-travel experience. Make sure you've agreed everything with your partner first (see page 138) or you might end up showing all to the world.

6. STILETTOS

We've already established the pros of high heels but for S&M they're essential to establish the power divide – no, not on him, he can just wear big boots. For you, they're sex armour, and the spikier, the better.

7. CAT O' NINE TAILS

A flick-y sort of whip, which swishes appealingly across the butt without causing too much agony in its wake. Also looks excellent with any form of PVC cat-woman costume you dare wear. What do you mean, you haven't got a sewing machine?

8. CORSET

Restraint, fetishism and a tiny waist – you'll have it all with a corset. True sex-goddess wear, few men can resist the erotic symbolism of tightly laced breasts and waist. Whether you keep it on for sex or let him untie you first, it's definitely worth the hassle of lacing it up in the first place.

9. PADDLE

Small hitting devices, which resemble ping pong bats, are ideal for the sadist who doesn't like to get her hands sore. Paddles enable effective bottom slapping from a short distance and make the job much easier because your arms won't get as tired – though his bottom might.

10. SILK SCARVES

Easier to untie than ropes, tape and handcuffs, silk scarves are failsafe bondage equipment. They undo very easily, they feel sensual and they also double up as blindfolds. Every home should have at least two, but make sure they've not got nylon in them or the knots will never come apart.

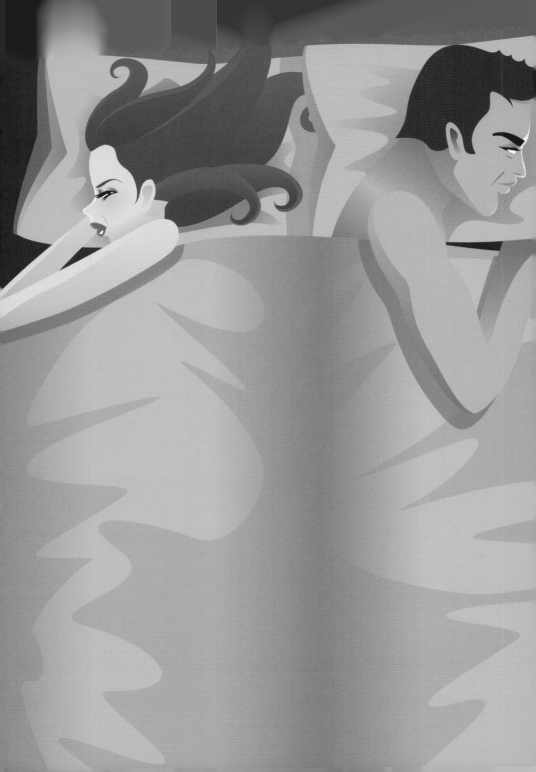

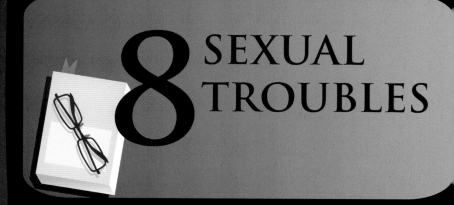

8 SEXUAL TROUBLES

'WHEN CHOOSING BETWEEN TWO EVILS I ALWAYS PICK THE ONE I NEVER TRIED BEFORE.'

MAE WEST

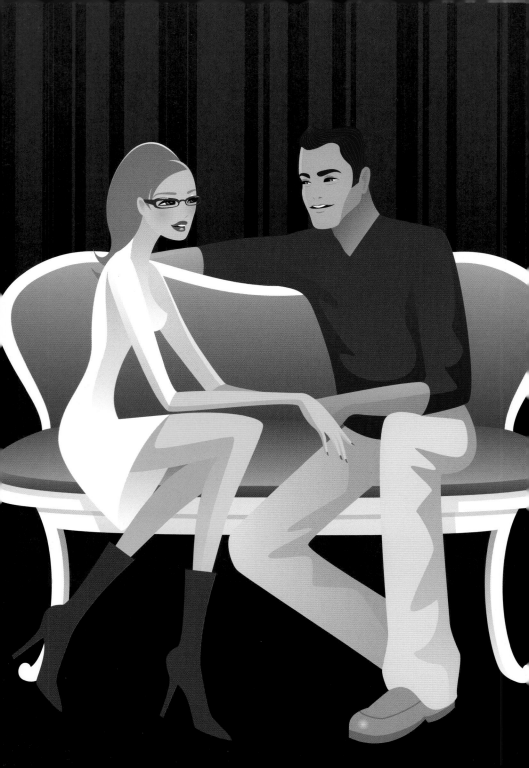

SEXUAL TROUBLES

Now, you've bravely ploughed through the entire book. By this time, you'll know how to ensnare a man at fifty paces and exactly what to do when you've got him. You'll know how to dress, how to move and what to say to take your deserved place as a qualified sex goddess. But there's just one problem and it's this: all the technical knowledge, attitude and beauty in the world will not give you a great sex life if you and your partner can't communicate.

Communication is the lifeblood of good sex; without it you can run through a repertoire of bedroom tricks that would startle a Bangkok hooker and nothing will flicker but the bedside light. Of course, most relationships start off with the communication highways running smoothly and congestion-free. But as time goes by, life gets in the way of love and work, tiredness, kids, socializing and bills, and DIY and TV begin to replace those hours you once spent sharing every last thought and emotion that passed through your mind. Admittedly, it may have been a pain for everyone else, but for you and him, it was bliss. Once those days are gone and you've thrown in a hefty sprinkling of resentment, unresolved annoyance, daily irritants, jealousy and marital martyrdom, it's a wonder you ever want sex at all. When you do, it's often perfunctory because no one wants to appear vulnerable or to voice all the issues that remain under the carpet. Even if it is loving, it can still be basic because you're exhausted and you've both got an early start the next morning.

No wonder communication suffers. And if sex is just a pale shadow of how it used to be, it's unlikely that your bodies have changed, or you've unaccountably forgotten how to touch each other. It's much more feasible that you've forgotten how to talk to each other and that's why you've both lost that lovin' feeling (and it's gone, gone, gone... whooo-ooh).

And then there are the other sexual problems – the ones nobody likes to talk about at all, however good their communication skills might be, such as sexually transmitted diseases (STDs). Or the constant hassle of finding a form of contraception that works and doesn't ruin sex or your mood. In fact, it's a wonder anyone has good sex at all when you think about it. But they do, and so can you, with a bit of insider knowledge.

HOW TO COMMUNICATE

Without 'emotional intelligence' you can't be a sex goddess. The term is simply a fancy description for empathy – the ability to understand how someone else is feeling and recognize your own feelings for what they are. We all know that depression is often unexpressed anger and that anger is frequently a disguise for fear, but remembering it when we're about to throw a plate at his head is the hard part.

So if communication has broken down to the point where sex seems an unwelcome intrusion into your life, the first thing you need to do is to sit down together to talk and listen. Built-up resentment between you usually means that one person expresses how they feel while the other interrupts, and the whole thing can end in a shower of recriminations and abuse, so you need to borrow a few tricks from relationship therapy.

To ensure that you both have a fair chance to talk without interruption, set a time limit during which one person speaks and the other is not permitted to interrupt, and then you swap over. (Use an egg timer so no one cheats.) Try not to make wild, sweeping generalizations such as 'you always' and 'you never'. Instead, try to restrict your explanations to how you feel. For example, rather than saying, 'You make me upset when…', accept that being upset is your own response and say, 'I feel upset when I feel unheard,' or something similar. Take the accusation out of the sentence and it is much easier to hear. You can also check that you've understood what you're being told by repeating his words back to him. Otherwise it's very tempting only to hear what you assume he's saying, and not the reality.

If your communication problems are largely confined to sex, take the pressure off by discussing them outside the bedroom. Practical sex problems are much easier to resolve than emotional issues, but both will be eased by communicating effectively. So if you don't like what he does in bed, remember that the golden rule is 'four pieces of praise to one piece of negativity'. Slot 'It hurts me when you get too rough and I don't like it' in among 'You're such a good kisser' and 'I love being in bed with you'. Try not to sound carping or weary. Imagine how you'd like to be asked to change your sexual behaviour and adapt your tone accordingly.

If he's criticizing you, ask yourself whether he has a point, but never accept personal abuse or cruelty. Anything he says should be asked or offered from a position of him loving you and wanting to improve your relationship. If you're not sure, ask yourself this question, 'If my best friend's boyfriend spoke to her like that, would I think he was being reasonable or would I regard him as a brute?' Most women, even sex goddesses, have a tendency to run themselves down, so don't aid and abet a bully by checking your self-esteem in at the door.

If your communication problems seem too severe to overcome, sexually or otherwise, consider counselling. Try couples therapy or one-to-one. While this may not make a silk purse of a sow's ear, it can be invaluable in helping you to decide whether to stay or go. In healthy relationships most issues can be resolved with a cunning combination of listening and compromising… just make sure you're not the only one doing either.

WHAT HAPPENS IF YOU GO OFF SEX?

Few women are constantly sex-mad. Hormones, periods, pregnancy, stress and tiredness can mess with the female sex drive as effectively as nuclear testing messes with nature. Occasionally going off sex doesn't mean you're not a sex goddess, more that you're normal. But the real problem arises when you go off it and stay off it. The likeliest explanation is that your feelings for your partner have changed and your sex drive will return in full flower when you meet someone new.

Other issues to look at include body image, both yours and his. For example, if he has recently put on a lot of weight or stopped exercising/displayed visible signs of ageing, he may feel less desirable and therefore stop making approaches. His altered appearance may also put you off, albeit subconsciously.

Equally, if you don't feel good about yourself, you won't feel like a sex goddess and every time you get naked, you'll be obsessing about your flab instead of enjoying the sensations and the closeness. Unfortunately, the media plays a large part in suggesting that no one can possibly be worth making love to unless they weigh less than a gnat and have a stomach you could bounce dried peas off.

But good sex has been continuing for many millennia. The human race has not died out yet, so it stands to reason that people found each other sexually attractive even when they had missing teeth and tanning only happened in leather workshops. So all you modern-day sex goddesses out there, remember just how desirable you are. Of course, if you are ill, exhausted, stressed and tense, or suffering from PMT (PMS), no one expects you to be having sex, though if you try it, you might surprise yourself. Then again, you might be happier simply being left in a corner with a box of chocolates and a DVD of *Breakfast at Tiffany's*.

Sometimes nothing you do helps you feel like having sex. If that's the case, you may be suffering from depression or even a hormonal imbalance. If your libido has packed its bags and gone away, seemingly for good, it's worth going to see the doctor. Unless your partner's suddenly put on lots of weight and refuses to wash, of course, in which case your lack of desire is perfectly understandable.

SEXUAL DISEASES

The fastest growth in STDs (sexually transmitted diseases), also known as STIs (sexually transmitted infections), is currently among young women, which suggests we're being less careful than we once were. Nobody's judging the number of sexual partners you may have had, but whoever you sleep with, whether it's one man a year, seventeen a week or just your husband, unless you have conclusive proof that they are not carriers or have never suffered any STDs, you'd be insane not to insist on using a condom.

A few mild mentions for the first two weeks of your relationship, followed by a drunken night of passion when you're sure it's safe and after which you don't bother any more, does not count as protecting your sexual health. Condoms are better than they used to be; they're thinner and more sensitive. Compare them with a month of discharge, uncomfortable itches and the abject terror that you've caught something unmentionable.

The good news is that so long as you're prepared to go and be examined, nearly all STDs can be cured with antibiotics or a painless procedure. But if you refuse to face up to your symptoms, you may risk such illnesses as pelvic inflammatory disease (PID), which can lead to infertility, not to mention the risk of passing it on to your partner and possibly all his future partners.

Needless to say, if you're having sex with a guy whose penis is not looking all that great – cracked skin, discharge or even spots – the chances are he's already contracted an STD and you should avoid him like the plague. However, many men are apparently symptom-less, or else he may have had something once and now he's just a carrier, which means he can pass it on without showing any signs. With a new partner, it's always hard to tell – and he may not know that he's a carrier. Which is why you should continue using condoms for at least six months to two years, which gives most diseases a chance to develop. If he's been exposed to HIV or hepatitis C, then he must get tested regardless.

CHLAMYDIA

Over half of those infected have no visible symptoms. In women, the bacteria affects your cervix and if you do show symptoms they may include yellowish discharge, bleeding or spotting between periods, and pain on urinating. This is a disease you must tackle, or it can lead to pelvic inflammatory disease, (PID). Antibiotics can be used to treat chlamydia, but you may have infected your partner(s), so you'll need to tell them too. Not fun, but essential.

CRABS

The familiar term for pubic lice, crabs are passed around in a similar way to head lice, only via pubic hair. They are visible and, although harmless, very itchy and unpleasant. Crabs can be treated with a special shampoo, but the itching may remain for up to two weeks after they've gone.

CYSTITIS

Although not sexually transmitted, cystitis is an inflammation of the bladder and/or urethra, often caused by rough sex, and is sometimes referred to as 'honeymoon' cystitis. The symptoms are a sensation of burning when you urinate, cloudy urine and the frequent need to pee, but then nothing happening when you get there. Drink plenty of water and cranberry juice, which is good for your bladder, but if it's really bad you'll need antibiotics to clear it.

GONORRHOEA

This is also known as 'the clap'. Women seldom display severe symptoms, but if you do, they resemble those of chlamydia, while men get soreness and discharge. This is one STD that can lead to pelvic inflammatory disease (PID) and infertility, so if you suspect you've taken a risk, you must take antibiotics and inform your partner of your situation. As with any sexually transmitted disease, do not have unprotected sex until your treatment is completed and the infection has cleared.

HERPES

Symptoms include blisters on your genitals, which will burst and form ulcers. The first attack can involve flu-like symptoms and blisters will be sore. Unfortunately, there's no cure; once the virus is in your bloodstream, it will lie dormant and recur occasionally. However, it can be managed, but you must visit a specialist. Avoid sex when the virus is active and use creams and antiviral drugs to minimize discomfort.

HIV

Lately, young men and women have become less fearful of contracting HIV (human immunodeficiency virus). The mass panic of the 1980s has become more of an afterthought for the next generation – but it shouldn't have. It's now spreading faster among straight women than gay men (because gay men got the condom message). The virus attacks immune cells in the body and quickly mutates, which means that normal infections can take hold and eventually develop into AIDS (acquired immunodeficiency syndrome). Modern drugs vastly improve life expectancy and life quality of sufferers, but the simplest way to avoid it is to use a condom.

SYPHILIS

The disease of nineteenth-century Paris has returned and is thoroughly unpleasant. You're unlikely to catch it, but just in case, symptoms include an initial genital ulcer, which enters your bloodstream and leads to further breakouts. In turn, this damages the immune system and, finally, the heart and brain. It can be cured via muscle-injected antibiotics; left untreated, it can kill you, so don't casually ignore that weeping genital ulcer, will you?

THRUSH

Also referred to as 'yeast infections', thrush is an infection of the candidiasis fungus, which can overpower your natural bacteria and cause symptoms that include itching, soreness around your vagina and a thick whitish discharge. It is not usually related to sex, though it can be spread via this route, including oral sex. Topical creams and pessaries, available over the counter from pharmacies, are the usual cure.

TRICHOMONIASIS VAGINATIS

This infection is due to a parasitical bacterium and results in a greenish discharge, an unpleasant fishy smell, and soreness and burning around the vulva. Sometimes there are no apparent symptoms. Again, antibiotics can sort it out.

WARTS

Caused by the human papilloma virus, genital warts are small, cauliflower-shaped growths around the labia and vagina. You catch them through contact with infected skin and they may take up to two years to develop. The warts can be treated with a chemical cream or frozen off.

CONTRACEPTION

There are so many forms of contraception available, you'd think remaining baby-free would be simple. However, nature wants you to get pregnant, so the only way to avoid its wishes is to be efficient when it comes to using your chosen method of contraception. Having it on the shelf will not prevent you getting pregnant, nor will carrying it in your purse. If you don't take note of the instructions, in nine months' time you'll be a sex goddess with a screaming bundle. Reading through the following options will help you to discover the method that suits you and your partner, best. Consult a medical professional for further advice.

CAP/DIAPHRAGM

Like condoms, these work via the barrier method, so they don't mess around with your hormones. Both versions fit inside your vagina, covering your cervix so that sperm can't penetrate. Diaphragms are rubber domes, but caps are generally smaller and made from silicone. The upsides are that you can put them in place well before sex, so there's no interruptions, and they can stay in for a while afterwards. However, you have to use them with spermicide, which can be messy, and they can be awkward to fit and take out of yourself. They will need to be refitted if your weight changes more than 4.5kg (10lb) and after giving birth. You will also need to inspect them for tiny holes and get them replaced periodically.

THE COIL/INTRAUTERINE DEVICE

The coil, or IUD, is a little copper and plastic device that is fitted into your womb by highly trained professionals. It has a thread attached, which remains at the top of your vagina and it can stay in place for three to ten years. Coils aren't generally recommended if you haven't had a child, and they can cause pain and heavy periods, but if you want a non-hormonal form of contraception that you can forget about, it's worth considering

COITUS INTERRUPTUS

Otherwise known as 'getting off the stop before', this involves the man pulling out before he ejaculates. All I can say is, that's how I got pregnant. Not a reliable method by any means.

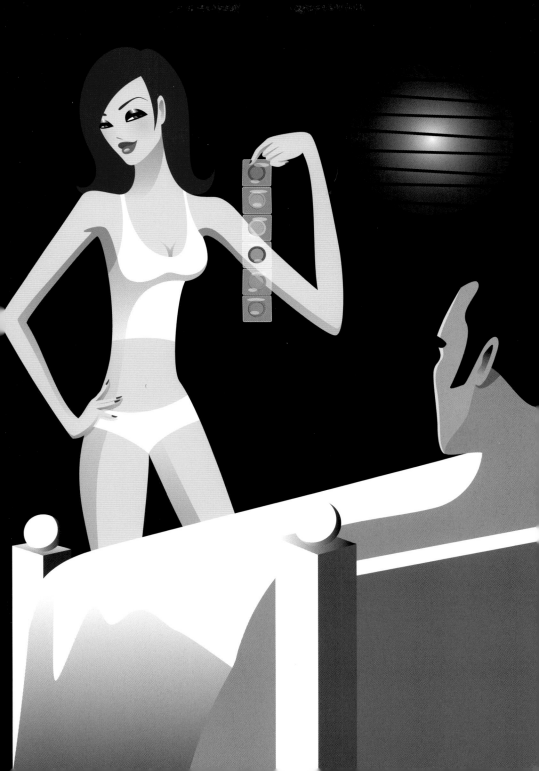

CONDOM/FEMIDOM

Condoms are remarkably simple yet effective – they stop the sperm entering your body and keep it all in a little bag. The downsides are that you have to halt what you're doing, grope about for the packet, fail to rip the plastic open, he may lose his erection, the light gets switched on and, eventually, you wonder why you're bothering. Still, they do work and, most vitally, they protect you from STDs. As for the Femidom, I've never met anyone who's used it more than once as it's like sticking a hooped crinoline up your vagina. But it is highly effective against pregnancy and STDs.

CONTRACEPTIVE IMPLANTS

Small flexible tubes are placed under the skin of your arm and release progesterone from year to year. Norplant and Implanon are currently available. Norplant is effective for five years and Implanon for three. Again, this is ideal if you're trekking through Borneo with no access to a drugstore, but there are reports of unpleasant side effects and many women have had them removed well before the time is up.

DEPO PROVERA

This is the progestogen-only injection, a long-term method that's ideal for the forgetful woman. Depo Provera (the most common type) protects you for up to three months, however there can be side effects such as mild depression. Because the hormone is injected into the muscle and is slowly released, you can't get rid of it for the entire time it's in you, so be very sure before you decide to take it.

MORNING-AFTER PILL

If you've had a broken condom (which is doubtless what you'll tell the nurse, even if you were just drunk and forgot to use anything), you can get emergency contraception known as the Morning-After Pill. There are two pills, containing a massive dose of hormones, which you take 12 hours apart. Chances are that you'll feel very sick. You can take it up to 72 hours after sex, but don't make a habit of it – it's really not good for you. In some countries it is available at pharmacies or from a general practitioner.

THE PILL: COMBINED

So-named because it combines the hormones progestogen and oestrogen, the Combined Pill stops your ovaries releasing an egg every month and it thickens your cervical mucus. It also thins your womb lining, making it much harder to accept a fertilized egg. Many women swear by the Pill as it is a nonintrusive barrier method. But if you're over 35 or a smoker, it's not a wise move, as it can raise blood pressure and increase the risk of strokes, among other problems.

THE PILL: MINI

The progestogen-only pill contains a hormone similar to one naturally produced in the ovaries. It's a milder dose than the Combined Pill because it simply thickens your cervical mucus to prevent an egg turning up unannounced. However, it's also slightly less reliable and you have to have a good memory because you have to take it at the same time every day.

RHYTHM METHOD

Beloved of hippies and Catholics, the rhythm method is noninterventionist and based on nature's cycles, which is why so many of its devotees have at least six children. In an ideal world, however, it works by teaching you to recognize your fertile and infertile times, by logging your daily temperature when you wake up and by understanding your cervical secretions – as if you've nothing better to do – and understanding the pattern of your menstrual cycle. There are electronic fertility devices, such as Persona, which can help, and these involve you urinating on sticks of paper and entering in data about your cycle. But, really, isn't it easier just to use a condom? After your period, you may notice a few days when you feel dry. No cervical secretions will be seen or felt. Then the secretions produced by your cervix change in texture and increase in amount. At first, they feel moist, sticky and white or cloudy. This is the start of the fertile time. The secretions then become clearer, wetter, stretchy and slippery, like raw egg white. This is a sign that you are ovulating and at your most fertile.

TOP TEN SEXUAL WORRIES AND HOW TO BEAT THEM

Sexual worries can ruin your life – but they don't need to. Nowadays it's easier than ever to get help, whether via the Internet, books, magazines or just talking to friends. There are clinics dedicated to sexual health that will not, I promise, judge you, and psychotherapists who specialize in sexual issues. So you don't need to suffer in silence.

1 CAN'T COME, WON'T COME

If you simply cannot orgasm, it's far more likely to be down to emotional, rather than physical, reasons. You may be scared of sex, afraid to let go and appear vulnerable, or you have learned from your upbringing that nice girls 'don't'. Talk to your partner, let him know just how patient he has to be and consider counselling. If masturbation doesn't work, it could be a physical problem and you'd benefit from seeing a doctor. Some women suffer from vaginismus, a condition where the vaginal muscles freeze to prevent entry. This does not mean you're frigid, just that you may need therapy to get to the root of the problem.

2 THE CONDOM QUESTION

'I didn't know how to mention it' is not a good excuse when you're suffering from a sexual disease that you could have avoided if only you'd used a condom. Deep down, all men know they should use one – and if he seems dismissive, doesn't mention it or, worse, refuses to have sex wearing one, then you really need to make it clear. Carry your own, don't rely on him, and make sure they're accessible at the crucial moment. A selection of different varieties to choose from can make wearing one a tiny bit more appealing. A calm 'I never have sex without one' should do the trick – and if not, ask yourself if you really want this man.

3 HE WANTS THINGS I DON'T

If your partner is pressurizing you to indulge in sexual practices that you hate, ask yourself what's going on. Do you dislike what he's suggesting because someone else told you it was bad, or because you genuinely know it's not for you? If the latter, any decent partner will drop the subject once you've given him an outright 'No'. However, if your reluctance extends as far as sex in any position but missionary and an aversion to blow jobs, then it's not entirely his fault and you may both benefit from a little couple counselling.

4 HE WANTS IT MORE THAN ME

Mismatched sexual appetites are a serious problem for many couples. But as Woody Allen said in *Annie Hall*, 'She never wants sex – maybe two, three times a week,' while Diane Keaton sighed, 'We do it all the time – twice a week at least.' So it's as much about perception as frequency. You may both have to compromise – let him take sexy pictures of you and masturbate over them, or give him a handjob instead, while he must accept that daily sex is a rare occurrence in most relationships, at least past the first month.

5 HE THINKS ABOUT HIS EX/PORN

Insensitivity is the enemy of good sex, not to mention good communication. So if your partner likes to remember the hot time he had with his ex, or remark on how stunning some babe walking down the street looks, he's committing the cardinal sin of relationships. Sexually speaking, this should be the bottom line: unless specifically asked, he may never refer to a previous partner's sexual habits. And of course, neither should you. If he does, say, 'Well, that was then, this is now,' and let him know that you find the gory details offputting and unsexy. That should shut him up.

6 SMALL PENIS

A penis that's genuinely classed as a micro-penis is under 5cm (2in), so I bet it's not that bad. The average for Caucasian guys is about 15cm (6in), Asians 12.5cm (5in) and if the guy's of African extraction 17.5cm (7in). And it's more or less true that it's what you do with it that counts. However, if it's very thin or short, you may have trouble enjoying all the wonderful sensations of sex. There's very little he can do about it, so be kind. Close your thighs when he enters you to narrow your vagina and squeeze your internal muscles around his penis – this is guaranteed to make a thin penis feel wider and it will increase the friction, and the resulting intensity of feeling, for the both of you. Remember you only have nerve endings in the first 7.5cm (3in) anyway, so so long as he can thrust, you can still have a good time.

7 HE'LL THINK I'M TARTY

Plenty of women, sex goddesses included, are convinced that if they speak their true desires to their partner, he'll leave them for someone more traditional. Women are still afraid of being seen as 'whores' if they want any kind of experimental sex that falls outside the normal boundaries of what 'nice girls do'. It's important to remember that you have just as much right as any man to state what turns you on, and to ask your partner to fulfil your desires. Bed is the place where you can truly be yourself and if you feel you can't, it may not be your needs that are wrong, but your partner's attitude. Although if you're demanding he dresses up as your ex, his reluctance may be understandable. He's sensitive too, so go easy on him.

8 PREMATURE EJACULATION

If the problem is two strokes and you're out, he may be suffering from premature ejaculation. He may be too excited, too nervous or too inexperienced to hold on (see pages 96–97 for techniques to calm him down). If the suggested methods don't work, it may be a symptom of a psychological problem, in which case he'll benefit from seeing a psychosexual counsellor to discuss his feelings about sex.

9 NEVER HAVE TIME FOR SEX

Life has a tendency to take over from sex and suddenly, by the time you've staggered through everything you have to do, the very idea of having any time for sex seems insane. In that case, you need to book time, just as you would for a meeting or a gym session. It may sound heartless and unromantic, but what's romantic about never having sex at all? Pencil in, for example, a Friday night, take a bottle of wine to bed and get down to it. You'll feel ten times better and you can make it a regular date in future.

10 BORED OF SEX

What if you are still attracted to him and still like him, but you just can't be bothered to have sex anymore? Basically, you've slipped into a rut and your libido has died. But it's not the end; there are ways to revive it, chief of which is to get out of the house. Environment plays a bigger part in sex than we realize and one night in a hotel room, away from all the demands of bills, kids and washing, can do wonders. Or try music, candlelight and a picnic on the living room floor. Buy new underwear, invest in a vibrator and rekindle your desire by thinking about what attracted you to him in the first place. With sex, it's a case of use it or lose it.

AFTERWORD

Congratulations! You are now a fully-fledged sex goddess, ready to hit the world with your charm, grace and sensuality. Be aware, however, that everyone has off days. No one feels like a sex goddess all the time and no one acts like one the whole time. But you can still use your inner sex goddess as a guide to how you should feel about yourself. All women deserve to feel desirable, confident and loved. Keep telling yourself that you are, keep acting as though you are, and you've pretty much cracked it. And if someone you love keeps telling you differently, it's their problem, not yours. The single most important thing for any sex goddess to remember is that she's worth it. Don't let anyone bring you down, because you deserve only the best, from life, love – and, of course, sex.

'You deserve only the best, from life, love – and, of course, sex.'

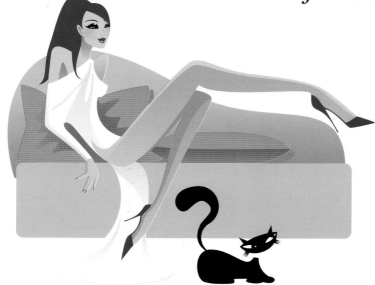

RESOURCES

Bibibaby
www.bibibaby.co.uk
Bisexual advice and meeting

Brook
www.brook.org.uk
Sexual health and contraception

Cake
www.cakenyc.com
Entertainment and parties

The Clitoris
www.the-clitoris.com
Female desire and fantasy, sex
techniques, health and more

Family Planning Australia
www.shfpa.org.au
Reproductive and sexual health

Female First
www.femalefirst.co.uk
Online magazine for women

Libida
www.libida.com
Sex toys, erotic books and
dvds, plus advice, health and
erotica

LoveHoney
www.lovehoney.co.uk
Toys, gifts, lubes and condoms
direct to your – or your lover's
door

Masturbate for Peace
www.masturbateforpeace.com
Sex toy shopping, poetry,
pictures and masturbation
resources

Nerve magazine
www.nerve.com
Ezine for online erotica

Planned Parenthood
www.plannedparenthood.org
Sexual health advice and family
planning

Salon
www.salon.com/sex
Ezine on sex, society, politics
and culture

Tabooboo
www.tabooboo.com
Online sex toys and shopping

QUOTATIONS

The publisher and author
would like to thank the
following sources for the
quotations that appear
throughout the book:

pages 9 and *24* Sophia Loren,
from *Halliwell's Filmgoer's
Companion*, Flamingo, 1984.

page 21 Raquel Welch, www.
classicscifi.com. 'Goodness…'
Mae West, as Maude Triplett in
the 1932 film *Night After Night*.
'I used to be Snow White' Mae
West, www.workinghumor.com.
Lauren Bacall, www.movie.
lifetips.com.

page 22 Lillie Langtry, from
*The Secret Sex Lives of Famous
People*, Chancellor Press, 1993.
page 23 Elizabeth Taylor,
www.celebritywonder.com.

page 24 Halle Berry, on
winning the Best Actress for
the film *Monster's Ball*, the
Academy Awards, March 2002.

page 25 Marilyn Monroe,
www.starspage.com.

page 27 Mae West, as Flower
Belle Lee in the 1940 film *My
Little Chickadee*.

page 43 Tallulah Bankhead,
www.geocities.com/holywood.

page 67 Mae West from *Mae
West on Sex, Health and ESP*,
W.H. Allen 1975.

page 85 Elton John, *Rolling
Stone Magazine*, October 1976

p*ages 105* and *123* Marilyn
Monroe, www.starspage.com

page 143 Mae West as Frisco
Doll in the 1936 film *Klondike
Annie*.

AUTHOR ACKNOWLEDGEMENTS
Thanks to S. Buckley for his useful insights into men, and to all my
lovely female friends, who don't need this book at all.